This book is a MUST-READ truly open your heart to love, s Jimmi-Ann is an extremely gi

~ **Amelia Aiken, cancer warrior-survivor**

My life was enriched by meeting Jimmi-Ann. You will never be the same after hearing her life story, and I am thrilled that she is sharing her experiences with a larger audience. You will definitely not want to let the parade pass you by after reading her book!

~ **Anne Gibson, fellow cast member for Hello, Dolly! and lifetime friend**

Jimmi-Ann and I were co-workers for many years. It was impossible to have a bad day when you worked across the hall, or even in the same building, as this woman! Her laugh, her smile, her warmth constantly radiating from her and spreading over to you. I am thrilled she took the time to share her story, not only to remind me of all the wonderful things about her but also to remind me of all the wonderful things about me. She is truly an inspiration.

~ **Susan Newton**

In this book, Jimmi-Ann describes how she conquered her fears and how the devastating diagnosis of cancer transformed her life. A story of faith, perseverance, fierce determination, and self-realization, her miraculous story is an inspiration to all.

~ **Pat Golus**

Jimmi-Ann Muse is a warrior! She has always been an inspiration to me, and this book just elevates her impact. She pushes herself to keep a positive focus even in the midst of the most challenging circumstances, and she knows to keep her eyes on the One who holds her every step of the way. Well done, Jimmi-Ann!

~ **Sara Fisher**

As a lifelong educator, Jimmi-Ann has dedicated her life to teaching. This book is a continuation of that passion as Jimmi-Ann takes the reader on a journey of learning, faith, healing, and resilience.

~ **Derick A. Pindroh, Executive Artistic Director— Foothills Playhouse—Jimmi-Ann's Former Student**

JA always put her positive attitude first. She's a true fighter who never gave/gives up! Cancer was no match for JA.

~ **Linda Stone**

I am anxious to read this book and anything from and about this amazing, creative, wonderful woman!

~ **Linda Grant**

Stage 4 to Center Stage! *is an amazing read that will give hope, coping mechanisms, healing, and love to the reader. She shares her story offering a path forward with complete healing in her life. Jimmi-Ann is a gifted writer, and her story will leave you feeling positive about whatever you are facing in your life!*

~ **Jim Aiken**

This very readable book will comfort you and encourage you with life experience, wisdom, and laughter should you ever need any of that. Its scenes of growth and joy would be especially powerful if you or someone you know must battle the dreaded "C word."

~ **Maxine Bennett**

This book illustrates how positive thinking and action are essential in every aspect of our lives and will open doors to miracles. The author is a powerful force of brightness dealing with a very real and dark health issue. She does it remarkably well and will hopefully inspire others to deal with any kind of upset in our lives. Good reading!

~ **Shannon Bledsoe**

Jimmi-Ann, in real life, is Dynamic, Loving, Loyal, Artsy, and hysterically Funny! So, it is no surprise that her book encompasses all these aspects of her personality and more. Real-life advice in a loving and spiritual way. Read it! You'll be inspired.

~ **Jeanne Dove**

Jimmi-Ann's journey through cancer required faith, tenacity, laughter, and love. Her story is both heartwarming and miraculous. In reading her account, Jimmi-Ann's wisdom and humor will reach into your life and encourage you to join with her in the magnificence of hope.

~ **Amenie Kristine Schweizer, Certified Holistic Health Practitioner**

A great, uplifting approach to what could have been a debilitating conversation. It's really about a state of mind. Jimmi-Ann Muse takes you from tears to mostly laughter through unleashed living eighteen years beyond the 'forecast' six months. Jimmi-Ann's big personality always keeps me in tears from laughing. Choosing that one person who continues to leave heartfelt impressions is Jimmi-Ann. A very joyful and inspirational read.

~ **Roxanne Koteles, Author, Food Coach**

Stage 4 to *Center Stage!*

Stage 4 to *Center Stage!*

*Cancer Conquered—
The Choice of Love Over Fear*

Jimmi-Ann Carnes Muse

Copyright © 2024 Jimmi-Ann Carnes Muse

All rights reserved. No part of this book may be reproduced by any mechanical, photographic, or electronic process, or in phonographic recording; nor may it be stored in a retrieval system, transmitted, or otherwise be copied for public or private use—other than for "fair use" as brief quotations embodied in articles and reviews—without the publisher's prior permission.

Published in the United States *by* Grass Feathers, LLC. Laurens, South Carolina
Edited by: Sheri Horn Hasan

ISBN (paperback): 979-8-9898903-1-6
ISBN (ebook): 979-8-9898903-2-3

Book design and production by www.AuthorSuccess.com
Cover art by istock.com

This book is dedicated to David, my soul companion, the mirror image of my heart, my husband. His love, compassion, encouragement, commitment, and strength never wavered. Combined with his extraordinary intelligence and unpredictable sense of humor, these qualities sustained me; they gave me the courage to listen to my heart, which permitted my spirit to ascend during my soul journey of discovery and self-realization. I am forever yours . . .

This book is also dedicated to the sister of my heart, my nurturing cheerleader, Barbara Shaw Brinson. She held my hand every day for seven months, ensuring that David and I were both swathed in compassion and the belief that all would be well. Barbara became my guiding light, leading me to a place where I could feel safe once again. I am eternally grateful . . .

Stage 4 To Center Stage *honors the memory of my parents, Marie Seeger Carnes and James Arthur Carnes, Jr. Their capacity for love and laughter became my first brilliant life lessons. I know that you are collectively rejoicing—celebrating my transformative journey. I am so very blessed to have been yours to nurture.*

CONTENTS

Introduction: An Invitation to Share My Journey   1
Cast of Characters   5
Prologue   7

ACT I: The Curtain Opens Launching My Miraculous Journey   9

Scene 1   11
A Horrifying Prognosis: *A Staggering Reaction*

Scene 2   18
Surgery: "We got it all!"— "Oops! Sorry, you're as good as dead!"

Scene 3   25
The Oncologist's Verdict: *Plot Twist! Sharing the Diagnosis Opens Doors to Miracles*

Scene 4   32
Radical Changes in My Wisdom Regarding Food: *Setting the Stage for Successfully Conquering the Disease*

Scene 5   41
Extraordinary Misadventure! Upon Reflection: *Grocery Store Calamity Becomes Comedic Episode!*

Scene 6   49
A New Life in the Kitchen: *Vegetables–Southern Manner of Preparation Strictly Prohibited!*

ACT II: Possibilities Multiply as Belief in Miracles Grow   57

Scene 1   59
Optimism Required: *Positive Thinking is Essential for Opening Doors to Miracles*

Scene 2   65
My Script for Vibrant Living: *The Warrior's Arsenal ~ Twenty-One Weapons for Survival and Victory*

Scene 3 — 78
Not Quite Ready to Believe: *Two More Miracles on the Road to Recovery*

Scene 4 — 83
Quantum Physics Annihilates the Inner Monologue: *The Gift of Self-Acceptance and Self-Love*

Scene 5 — 90
Building Blocks for My Wall of Hope: *Timelines, Affirmations, and Prophesies*

Scene 6 — 96
It's All About Perspective: *Chemotherapy is Not a Wake or a Funeral!*

Scene 7 — 103
Road Trip the Day After My First Chemotherapy Treatment: *A Most Significant Pathway to Recovery is Revealed*

ACT III: Embracing the Richness of a Life-Transformed — 111

Scene 1 — 113
An Emergency Hospital Visit: *Letting Go Becomes Another Lesson in Placing Myself First*

Scene 2 — 121
Overjoyed! I Get My Kid Fix! *Teaching One Class Each Week Recharges My Spirit*

Scene 3 — 125
My Warrior's Arsenal Proves Victorious: *Happy Halloween, Happier Thanksgiving, Happiest Christmas Ever!*

Scene 4 — 133
A Strong, Powerful New Me: *Angered by a Third Surgeon, I Invent the Cancer Patch!*

Scene 5 — 138
Another FoodWisdomRx™ Experience: *An Adventure in Fasting to Encourage Post-Chemo Toxin Elimination*

ACT IV: The Curtain Closes Only to Re-Open to   **147**
Spectacular Ever-New Beginnings

> **Scene 1**   **149**
> *Hello, Dolly!*—Living in Bliss—*Before the Parade Passes By!*
>
> **Scene 2**   **158**
> How I Have Changed: *Several Years Later . . .*
>
> **Scene 3**   **164**
> Blesséd Exultation: *The Magic of Being Love!*
>
> **Epilogue**   **175**
>
> **Appendix A**   **176**
> Life Lessons: Stage 4 to Center Stage!
> *A Guide to Lessons Learned*
>
> **Appendix B**   **183**
> Condensed Adaptation: The Warrior's Arsenal:
> *Twenty-One Weapons for Survival and Victory*

Resources   **189**
Endnotes   **192**
Acknowledgments   **194**

INTRODUCTION
An Invitation to Share My Journey

Suddenly shattered by a cancer diagnosis that promised death, I embarked upon a soul venture in defiance of the disease. With my husband David's unfailing support and an enormous cast of compassionate champions, I began to recognize pathways of opportunity as I strode bravely into the arena of possibility.

Professing to be too busy to exercise, I was overweight. My adrenal system, out of whack for a dozen years, was completely wrecked. Arthritis contributed to my fitness decline, also helping set the stage for the villainous carcinoma to invade.

Filled with love for everyone, blessed with an incredibly marvelous marriage, a loving family, and an ocean of friends, my life looked to be sublime. Life *was* wonderful—until I slowed down and had time to think about myself. A capable actress, I hid from others the feelings of inadequacy that had plagued me for years and years. I came to believe that a self-disapproving mindset contributed significantly to the deterioration of my well-being. I share my story about how I released myself from doubts, fears, and thoughts of not being worthy with the hope that others will be moved to do the same.

Teaching life skills through drama and art was a twenty-four/seven profession. A passionate over-achiever who rarely used the word *no*, I happily took on extra projects. My obsession with, and attention to, the most minute detail created more work—especially since I wrote most of the plays I produced.

I always strived for perfection in everything, especially myself—never believing, until Cancer opened my eyes, that I was perfectly created and already more than I ever imagined myself to be.

At my school, the drama teacher takes on every role in production. Besides imparting knowledge and directing, I design and build sets, costumes, props, lighting, and makeup; I also handle publicity. Although these elements of a theatrical event provide a wonderful, creative outlet, they are nevertheless time-consuming and exhausting, leaving me with less time for negative monologues to echo through my brain. Overworked because I thrive on challenges, my compulsion to *overdo* undoubtedly contributed to my deteriorating health.

Suddenly, *the* cancer diagnosis took away all this busy-ness, and I was forced to embark on an incredible journey of self-realization and self-awareness. If it was time for me to go, I was prepared; the universe was unfolding as planned, but I realized I needed to slow down and take care of myself.

I stubbornly refused to go without a fight! I resolved to take on the role of Warrior-Woman to conquer the debilitating disease! Although I believed Cancer to be a horrifying villain, through my experiences, I began to listen to my intuition and take direction from my more loving inner voice as Cancer also became the catalyst for evolutionary change and recovery. I became aware of precious life offerings I had been oblivious to in my rush!

It took a terminal diagnosis for me to appreciate that true richness is the *life* we are gifted!

When diagnosed, I heard myself declare that not only would I conquer this villainous adversary, but I'd help others because of my experience! Paralyzed with fear, I still heard Spirit speak through me. Somehow, I held on to that immediate response and soon began to believe it. It's my most sincere wish that my story provides hope

INTRODUCTION

and encouragement for others to wage war against this disease and helps them defeat it!

As a drama teacher, playwright, actress, and celebrated drama queen, I decided to create the spotlight for my narrative as I stepped forward to engage in the battle of my life! I chose Life over Death and destroyed the antagonist! Instead of writing chapters, I adhered to a theatrical theme and wrote this book in acts and scenes. The four acts are named as follows:

Act One: *The Curtain Opens: Launching My Miraculous Journey*
Act Two: *Possibilities Multiply as Belief in Miracles Grow*
Act Three: *Embracing the Richness of a Life-Transformed*
Act Four: *The Curtain Closes Only to Re-Open to Spectacular Ever-New Beginnings*

I identified sixty-five important *Life Lessons* as I waged war on Cancer. Hopefully, you'll be inspired to learn from them; a guide is provided at the back of this book. I also included an abbreviated version of *The Warrior's Arsenal*, which I built of twenty-one weapons to fight ill health. It doubtlessly helped me conquer Cancer and my feelings of unworthiness. This resource may be applied to situations where you need support for well-being or help to pull out of despair or grief. My armaments for wellness are also an effective way to approach living consciously.

My book also reveals significant nutritional changes essential to my recovery. Plus, I share affirmations for inspiration, encouragement, and comfort taken from my *Wall of Hope*. Many stories are woven throughout and help illustrate the sequence of events that resulted in defeating this disease; surprisingly, many are amusing.

I discovered that miracles are ours for the taking—if we learn to recognize and accept them! I now identify coincidences as *God-Incidences* because they become seeds for miracles. Embracing

Self-Love was essential to my quest for wellness, fitness, joy, and gratitude. God *is* Love, and I believe individuals are placed on this planet *to love*. I had given my affection away, saving little for myself. Surprised to learn that unconditional loving of self generates an endless flow, I now believe that self-value is integral to wellness. I would be thrilled if my story enriches your life. And I am blissfully grateful to be alive and well eighteen years after defeating the dreaded disease.

My soul journey is not a one-size-fits-all plan, it is mine alone. In sharing my story, I hope to inspire others to live their fullest lives, open their hearts wide, and feel the exhilaration of *being* Love. For me, cancer was a physical, emotional, and spiritual experience; I would not change a single moment. Miracles are accessible! Step into the arena of love and possibility to welcome astonishing revelations, blessings, and delights!

CAST OF CHARACTERS
In order of appearance

Protagonists: The Good Guys

Jimmi-Ann: Woman sentenced to death
Warrior-Woman: Jimmi-Ann's internal heroic fighter spirit
God/God-Voice/Spirit: Jimmi-Ann's intuition, guidance, and divine messenger
God-Incidences: Pathways to miracles
Love/Self-Love
David: Jimmi-Ann's loving and supportive husband
Barbara: Jimmi-Ann's best friend, champion, and caregiver
Roxanne: Food coach
Renée Brigman: Bearer of hope
Emilie: Renée's mother—*a cancer warrior*
Amenie: Jimmi-Ann's friend, energy healer/life coach
Gary Ellison: David's friend and confidante
Doc: Jimmi-Ann's compassionate oncologist
Nurse #1: Positive helper
Jim: Barbara's husband
Rosie: Roxanne's sister—*also a cooking specialist*
The Big Boss: Grocery store manager
Claude Austin: Jimmi-Ann's grandson
Derick Pindroh: Jimmi-Ann's former student
James Hall: Jimmi-Ann's son-in-law
Meg Coffey: Jimmi-Ann's co-worker
Surgeon #4: A competent, caring orthopedist
Former Student's Parent: Doctor
Wendy Coburn: Jimmi-Ann's former student

STAGE 4 TO CENTER STAGE!

Commander Warrior-Woman's Legion of Soldiers

Peace Gratitude Joy Hope Positivity Intuition Life
Optimism Prayer Food Acceptance Wisdom Grace
Trust Easiness Blessing Jubilation Faith Possibilities
Opportunities Compassion Belief Delight Wellness Fitness
Strength Revelations Thankfulness Determination

Antagonists: The Bad Guys

Cancer: The villainous destroyer
General Chaos: Usurper of Jimmi-Ann's world
Surgeon #1: Arrogance personified
Surgeon #2: Understudy for Surgeon #1
Surgeon # 3: The churlish doctor who motivates Jimmi-Ann to take further action

General Chaos' Minions

Death Doubt Fear Sorrow Distress Worry Trouble
What Ifs Unworthiness Anxiety Foreboding Grief
Anger Stress Defeat Guilt Blame Resentment Adversity
Self-Criticism Turbulence Worthlessness Inadequacy Misery
Self-Pity Resistance Surgery

Extras

Family Friends Colleagues Students General Practitioner
Elderly Lady Buzz Shopkeeper Stock Boy Innkeeper
Lay Preacher Emily Audrey Chemotherapy Enema
Retreat Cleric Receptionist Anita Nurse #2 Amelia
Anthony Nurse Practitioner Internist Tiffany DuPuy

PROLOGUE

"David, with you as my protector, how can I help but thrive? Your love, goodness, and strength embrace and uplift me. As we negotiate this drama together, we'll flourish. You always catch me whenever I fall and make my heart sing—
I love you completely!"
~ JIMMI-ANN

David A. Muse

When we first heard the doctor's diagnosis, I "grayed out," overcome by the heavy g-load on my psyche. Just before melting into an incoherent blob of protoplasm, Jimmi-Ann's voice slammed me forcefully back into the realm of the living with a resounding *"No!"*

At that moment, *I knew.*

This book is the result of the powerful culmination of determined, focused effort. Difficult? Certainly. Hardships serve to remind us that nothing worth having is ever just given. We must believe. Believe in God, believe in yourself, believe in others, and don't doubt the outcome. Jimmi-Ann found strength she had no idea she possessed and passed some on to me. I am so fortunate to have been witness to the following account . . .

ACT I

THE CURTAIN OPENS LAUNCHING MY MIRACULOUS JOURNEY

SCENE 1
A Horrifying Prognosis:
A Staggering Reaction

"Breathe! Breathe! Breathe! Good gracious,
alive, don't stop breathing!"
~ JIMMI-ANN

At age fifty-two I was given a death sentence due to my health on June 7, 2005. I was diagnosed with Stage 4 colon cancer. After a routine colonoscopy, it was revealed that cancer had metastasized to six tumors in my liver and multiple lymph nodes—in six months, I'd be dead. Statistically, I might live two years with the prescribed drug regimen.

"How long will I be on chemotherapy?" I ask.

"For the rest of your life."

Sound stops and movement ceases as the world momentarily stands still. I become simultaneously petrified, horrified, devastated, and bewildered upon hearing that single word: *CANCER*.

The crashing negativity it conveys erupts within my soul. My heart stops, breath ceases, and brain becomes immediately tormented by every dreadful cancer story I've ever heard. My imagination runs rampant and triggers Fear, Agony, and Rage. General Chaos appears, larger than life, awaiting Cancer's orders. His minions, behind him, anxious to charge at his command, are prepared to do battle!

But somewhere inside me, a mighty warrior awakens, ready to harness my fear, move through the dreadfulness, and get on with living.

"*No!*" I forcefully declare.

Although in shock, my mouth opens, and these words fall out: "*Thank God we know what's wrong with me. Now I can do something about it. This is going to be the best thing that ever happened. I'm going to come out of this better than ever, and I'm going to be able to help other people because of it!*"

I *know* that I spoke from God—from Divinity—from my soul, for in retrospect, I cannot imagine having that kind of courage in such a devastating moment.

"She's right, doctor," interjects David, my heart, my greatest friend, my husband of twenty-two years. "She was a premature baby who weighed under two pounds and wasn't supposed to live. She's been a fighter all her life—she'll beat this, too!"

We drive home in silence, supporting and loving each other, our hands clasped, overwhelmed with Sorrow but enfolded in Love.

The twelve months that follow are staggering as I'm propelled on a journey of self-awakening and self-realization I'd initiated many times before but always abandoned as the chaotic world intruded. I understand that there should be a balance of mind, body, and soul, but I've been too busy to take good care of myself for years.

I aspire to be perfect—an impossible dream—therefore, it's no surprise that I often engage in relentless self-criticism. Others know nothing about my feelings of unworthiness, for I am a skilled actor.

Suddenly forced into a life-or-death circumstance, it's either get your act together, Jimmi-Ann, or it's time to bring the curtain down.

I'll do it tomorrow excuses are wrenched from me; I begin to learn to live in the present. The *could haves* and *should haves* do not carry meaning, and the realization that time is precious holds the utmost significance. No longer is my refrain, "As soon as I do this, I will do that."

Now, I set out to learn how to be free—free to live a more genuine life without persistent guilt and self-deprecation, without worrying how others might perceive me. Although once a proverbial Peter Pan, I'd veered off course, and my authentic self was quietly lurking in the shadows. Little did I know of the adventures to come, as unbeknownst to me, my journey would turn into a character study of self-discovery and enhanced self-awareness. But I'm getting ahead of myself.

Forced to take time off from teaching as a master teacher with twenty-seven years of experience, it breaks my heart to take a sabbatical and leave my students. But the school community supports my decision to stay home and get well. Head of the Arts Department, I teach theater, visual arts, and a Multiple Intelligence class at Camperdown Academy, a school for children with dyslexia in Greenville, South Carolina.

The year I take to heal helps me develop in astounding ways, and I grow better able to serve myself, my family, my students, and my world once my metamorphosis manifests.

After the diagnosis, I set goals for myself and designed a timeline for healing. I have come to believe that change must come from within. Always my own harshest critic, I learn to cultivate compassion for myself. I dare to live in the present and begin to act as if what I yearn for has already happened while being grateful.

I begin to listen to my intuition and follow the path along which I'm being led. I believe that intuition is my God-Voice directing my life's journey. Spirit communicates with us often, but we don't always take the time to listen in our demanding, hectic lives.

Life Lesson #1: *Life's journey of discovery is ever-changing and never-ending; it requires persistent attention and nourishment.*

I discover that there are no coincidences; they are more appropriately named, for me, *God-Incidences*. God-Incidences are gateways to Miracles.

Life Lesson #2: *Miracles happen continually; if we pay attention, we become aware of them.*

Lines from Max Ehrmann's poem, the *Desiderata*, become my mantra. His advice about not worrying or imagining terrible outcomes is just what I need to help me begin to release Fear. His words help encourage me to open up to loving myself by confirming that I am as precious as meadows, evergreens, and heavenly spheres. David and I share Ehrmann's philosophy that the acknowledged and the unknown are developing as intended and that being in harmony with God is fundamental to a peaceful life. The reminder his lines evoke helps us cope with the turmoil Cancer creates in our world. He also recommends being cheerful, something I strive for throughout my journey.

However difficult it is to believe those words, I focus on the ideas they represent. Peace, gratitude, and joy take root in my heart in small increments and grow steadily. I'm directed by God and feel Him as my constant companion. Initially, I worry that asking for what I need is egotistical, but the miracles start immediately *precisely because* I am asking.

Life Lesson #3: *God wants us to ask for what we desire.*

Somehow, I hold on to the surprising optimism I'd demonstrated when presented with the diagnosis. And everything I *need* shows up.

I always teach my students that attitude is fundamental to maturity, growth, and development. *It's all attitude in the way that you walk* are lyrics to a song in one of my plays. As it suggests: *You take control, yeah, you're in control. People judge others by their attitude. It's all up to you to set up the mood.*

I recognize intuitively that I must take control of the situation and find the faith to believe I'll be shown the way. It's time for me to practice what I preach!

ACT 1 SCENE 1

Life Lesson #4: *We have the power to choose how we feel, so work to stay positive.*

Our culture has canonized medical professionals and often takes as gospel words uttered by these erudite demigods. I would not be writing this memoir if I had opened fully to my prognosis and accepted it as true. I believe that physicians need to be cautious with their words and should always provide the gift of hope no matter how bleak the diagnosis. It's one thing to speak from my soul, like a warrior, to proclaim that Cancer is the best thing that ever happened, but another altogether to hold onto that perspective.

The doctor's perception of reality keeps creeping in. Fear and Doubt inevitably surface. The words *terminal cancer* flash in my brain like a neon sign—I can't escape the constant reminder that I have this dreaded disease and am supposed to die.

My principal concern is for David. I choose to be strong for him because it's unbearable to see him worry. He fills my heart with joy, promise, pride, gratitude, and an everlasting contentment that illuminates the precious gift of love—transcending time and space. He has held my heart since we met; however, that is an entirely different story.

We do not reveal that *the* cancer has reached the deadliest level unless asked. I do not want my children, family, friends, or students to be overly concerned, so I act my heart out. "Don't be so anxious; everything will be okay. I feel good. I'll be fine."

Those who know and understand that this is an incurable disease play along with me; those who don't know believe my award-winning performances. Amazingly, before long, I summon the strength to believe them myself.

Nevertheless, Fear and Doubt set me into action. I begin clearing out our home, packing things up, labeling boxes, and giving much away—so that David will not be so burdened after I transition.

Interestingly, our house doesn't feel right; it feels desolate. The warmth, charm, laughter, and magic that permeate our household is dying. However, I refuse to live in a place with the ambiance of a mausoleum. I begin to put stored treasures back to recreate our precious sense of home. Maybe I will stay. Perhaps I can stay—*can I?* Can I find the courage to hold on to my beliefs?

I begin to actualize words I've heard since childhood: *When God does something dramatic in your life, when he takes something from you, He is not punishing you. He is just preparing you for something better.* God is Love. God is not harming me. Belief begins to take root. After all, I'm not dead yet. Even though I'm diagnosed as terminal, my days become much, much easier when I choose to truly believe and implement this fundamental philosophy.

I also begin to welcome each day with positive intentions and choices. One important choice I make is never to personalize the illness; I always refer to it as *the* cancer and never claim it. It takes hard work and dedicated focus to consistently stay in a positive space. While it's human to slip into negativity and despair, I live in good energy more often than not with single-minded determination and the help of my incredibly supportive network.

Life Lesson #5: Every day of your life is a gift and should be embraced with gratitude, love, hope, and joy.

One thing I hesitate about is spending money on consumables. My athletic shoes are in sad shape. How can I justify buying an expensive new pair of sneakers when I might not be around long enough to break them in? David encourages me to buy new shoes and several other items, which lessens my sense of guilt. I can't seem to stop my brain from being practical. It appears to be a simple thing, but when he encourages me to buy an expensive basket for my organic food purchases, I know, in the deepest part of my heart, that I *will* be around to use it.

To this day, I cannot look at that basket without smiling and feeling the engulfing tenderness I experienced when he said: "Go ahead, you want it. Get it. You'll use it for ages!" Seemingly an insignificant comment, but oh, so important when we are terrified about our uncertain future! David's belief in me and our continuing time together is essential to my healing.

Of course, my husband is acting for me as much as I'm acting for him. I agonize about his stress, and since men generally don't like to talk about their problems, assume he isn't discussing his grief with anyone. It's exhaustingly difficult for both of us to cope. Of course, he's stressed—the poor man looks as if he's been hit by a train.

I place my heart in his hands, and he cares for it exquisitely. He never once lets me down; he never falters. His devotion and care keep me from crumbling and give me the strength to face each new day. It may sound cliché, but David is the mate of my soul, and I breathe easier and feel whole when we're together. We are thankful for every moment we're alive on this glorious planet and choose to live united in light, love, and laughter.

SCENE 2

Surgery: "We got it all!"— "Oops! Sorry, you're as good as dead!"

> "Ninety-nine percent of the world's population are idiots."
> ~ GARY ELLISON

My story begins near midnight on December 23, 2004, when I become so violently ill that I lose Christmas Eve and Christmas Day. We believe it's food poisoning, but when I visit my family physician on December 27, she discovers I've contracted a viral infection. I'm placed on a round of antibiotics and feel much better within a few days.

Nevertheless, my doctor believes it's wise for me to follow up with a colonoscopy. When she asks if I prefer a female instead of a male to administer the procedure, giggles bubble forth because I think that a woman with delicate hands and a gentle touch is a much better choice.

There are only two female diagnostic gastroenterologists in the area, and the first available appointment is in mid-May. So, I decide to wait five and a half months for the examination since my situation isn't considered urgent. I've never experienced a colonoscopy and don't mind the delay. Perhaps it will give me time to get used to the idea. Once again, my imagination takes flight! I remember every unpleasant story I've ever heard relating to colonoscopy assessments.

I understand that refusing to get one—or any medical test, for that matter—out of fear or embarrassment should never be part of the decision process. In retrospect, should I have waited months for a female doctor to care for my health?

Yes, for I am where I am supposed to be, doing what I am supposed to do at this very moment. The darkest time of my life proves to be the most enlightening. I would not change it.

Life Lesson #6: *If we allow fear to be a motivating factor in our lives, then we never truly live.*

The colonoscopy is painless, and the preparation isn't the nightmare I had feared. *I advise everyone to be proactive about your body and do whatever you can to promote good health. Don't put it off! If you have a family history of colon problems, are forty-five years old, or suffer from digestive distress, please make an appointment to see your friendly, local gastroenterologist—male or female!*

I kissed David and underwent the procedure on May 15, 2005. I recall nothing of the examination and feel quite pleasant as I emerge from the anesthesia. Relaxed but a bit groggy, I am fine as I'm wheeled into recovery. We're informed that three small pre-cancerous polyps were removed—they're nothing to worry about. Together, we sigh a tremendous breath of relief.

Then comes dreadful news: A growth about the size of a grape needs to be excised, and I should see to that as soon as possible. I schedule an appointment for a surgical evaluation later that week. We meet the specialist with high expectations, innocently assuming everything will go well. He determines that surgery is necessary and sends me for x-rays so he can further analyze my situation.

The following week, my stomach is cut like a zipper from my belly button down, and nine inches of colon, along with multiple lymph nodes, are removed. I get out of bed on the day of surgery and walk down the hall several times, much to the surprise of the nursing staff. Previous surgeries proved that the more rapidly one moves after an operation, the easier the recovery.

Later in the day, the surgeon assures us he "got it all." We're elated! I suddenly become aware that I'm *breathing*.

Much later, I realize this surgery is a blessing in disguise, a God-Incidence that prompts several beneficial lifestyle changes to help me get into better physical shape. (As you will learn, it postpones the chemotherapy treatments for eight weeks to allow for healing. God gives me seven weeks to eat the right foods and ease into exercising to get my body into tip-top shape to deal with the chemicals I'll be given.)

Life Lesson #7: *Perceived tragedy can evolve into the greatest of blessings.*

The next encounter with the surgeon proves devastating. He apologizes for the encouraging news at the previous evaluation but tells us that the removed lymph nodes *are malignant*, and *the* cancer has metastasized to my liver!

His radiologist had written up the tests before surgery as Stage 3, noting that carcinoma had spread into the liver. I gather that the surgeon never reviewed the radiologist's report, believed he had removed all the diseased cells during surgery, made his buck, and sewed me up without ever looking at the assessment.

While glad that this chunk of poison has been taken out of me, we're devastated at this shocking reversal of fortune! The cancerous lymph nodes removed during the surgical procedure mean the malignancy is now at Stage 4, the deadliest phase.

With six tumors spread throughout my liver, I need to see an oncologist. The surgeon's receptionist makes an appointment with a local cancer specialist, but I must wait six weeks to see him. Frustrated at this delay, my general practitioner secures an appointment for me to be seen by a noteworthy professional the following week in another town. This esteemed, popular oncologist has a very long waiting list, yet somehow, I miraculously become his patient without delay. This was another of the astonishing God-Incidences gifted to me during my journey!

My general practitioner also sends me to consult with a nutritionist. He recommends certain herbs and supplements and teaches me several relaxation techniques that I employ throughout the journey—especially when Fear rises to terrorize. His guidance and knowledge ease my heart and remind me of the value of releasing Guilt through Forgiveness. Our work and conversations are important early components that promote peace of mind—and, hopefully, my ultimate recovery.

Life Lesson #8: Embrace a loving and forgiving spirit; make every effort to be at ease and delight in the gift of life.

I do not return to work after my surgery because it's near the end of the school year. Plus, at that early date, I'm zombie-like when I'm alone. Facing students on a daily basis with the burden of Cancer suffocating me is too shattering to contemplate. To act like all is well when I'm around others is exhausting.

Graduation is, of course, a highlight of the school year. I can't attend commencement exercises due to my surgery, so David delivers my congratulatory speech for a graduating eighth grader in my stead. Best friend, husband, lover, confidant, personal assistant, and now public speaker—is there anything this man won't do for me?

I prayed for years to die before David because the thought of life without him was unbearable. Now, I thank God for answering my prayers, but tell Him that I have changed my mind!

Life Lesson #9: *Be careful what you ask for because God wants to provide!*

Several days after the colon surgeon's devastating report, I'm scheduled to have my bandages changed at his office. While sitting in the waiting room, I ask for a sign that everything will be well. I'm not ready to leave my husband; we still have things to accomplish in this lifetime, and I want to know how long he and I will be together. Suddenly, at that *precise* moment, I hear the sweet voice of an elderly patient behind me:

"David and I have been together for sixty-three years. Today is our anniversary."

My ears perk up and my heart swells. *Whoa!* This is no coincidence! This is my sign: A direct line from heaven, assuring me we will have more years together.

The doctor who performed my surgery is away, or maybe too embarrassed to face me, so his colleague checks my incision and removes the bandages to find that some of the external sutures have pulled out.

"The inside stitches are holding, but you should get a girdle to hold yourself together," he tells me.

For some unfathomable reason, I focus on the word *girdle*. Now, I haven't worn a girdle since the 1970s and haven't, thank goodness, even seen one since then! I ask, thinking *girdle* might be a term for a particular medical product. "Where do I find one?"

He snidely replies, "Belk's . . . JCPenney's . . . the girdle store."

Not yet stymied by his sarcasm, I plow on to ask if I should worry about the incision.

"Only if your guts fall out," he replies.

I nearly fall off the table.

David and the nurse roll their eyes, clearly not amused.

"I beg your pardon?"

ACT 1 SCENE 2

"If your guts fall out over the weekend, just hold them in and go to the emergency room,"

Now, there have been very few times in my life when I've been rendered speechless—*this* is definitely one of them!

Seeing the incredulous look on my face, he says, "It could happen. Don't worry about it," Just hold them in and get to the emergency room."

He leaves.

The room falls completely silent.

I eventually gasp. "Did he really say that?"

"Yes," the nurse responds, "but don't worry. It won't happen." She grins, shakes her head, and murmurs: "He needs to work on his bedside manner."

"Ya think?"

She then tells us where to obtain a wide elastic band that will work in lieu of a girdle, be more comfortable, and cost less, too. She also tells us that I'll need my incision cleaned and packed daily and asks if there's someone who can provide that service . . . .

Oh yuck!

Oh no!

David?

My sweetheart wiggles his eyebrows suggestively and says he'd be happy to *play doctor*, which makes us laugh. He claims some such experience from when he was in the army, and I know he's bluffing. But I adore him all the more because now he's taking on the role of Florence Nightingale. In time, he'll prove that he can assist me in several areas where I experience limitations because of my open incision. He even becomes proficient at shaving my legs—and is surprised to learn ladies shave up our legs instead of down!

We hustle off to get the elastic band but, unfortunately, find only a size small in stock. However, since it's the weekend and I don't want to lose any guts, David and I venture into the store's restroom with permission and manage to haul me into that band!

We giggle and laugh and *streeeeeeeeeeeetch* that belt! It's a definite challenge to breathe as I'm so tightly encased! Gleefully, we meet our goal of avoiding spilt entrails and emergency rooms!

I still shiver when I recall that doctor and his disconnect with patients.

Life Lesson #10: *If you expect respect, it is essential to respect others!*

Family, friends, and co-workers are dear . . . they make dinners and deliver them daily or indulge us with treats and flowers. One well-wisher friend took to her bed after a day of deep spring cleaning for us; she'll always be held in my heart for her thoughtfulness and expertise as our impromptu housekeeper.

We're provided with unlimited support and hugs. Students and their parents come to visit, bringing homemade cards and tokens of affection. I smile and assure them that I will be well . . . all the while hoping, with all my heart, that this will be true. My performance—as well as David's performance—continues to be stellar for our family and friends as well as each other.

Nevertheless, Fear is always lurking, and Doubt often raises its serpent's head. I work consciously at staying positive as much as possible.

Soon, I'll meet with the very much sought-after oncologist. His group practice is located in a city fifty miles from our home. Incredibly, he has a satellite office in our town. His practice is one of five clinics in the U.S. associated with M.D. Anderson Cancer Research and Development Clinic out of the Houston Medical Center.

What were the chances of my long-distance oncologist having facilities so close by? It's a blessing—another surprising God-Incident!

SCENE 3

The Oncologist's Verdict:
Plot Twist! Sharing the Diagnosis Opens Doors to Miracles

"Jimmi-Ann needs a sign, Lord."
~ BARBARA BRINSON

David's holding my hand as we receive the ultimate crushing blow: Six tumors are spread throughout my liver, the largest the size of a golf ball. Since the growths are spread out, and in multiples, surgery is not an option. The oncologist reads the original PET scan for us, pointing out that the images show only one sign of activity—in the liver.

Since the PET and CT scan evaluations reflect activity in that organ, he believes *the* cancer has metastasized there and sees physical evidence that it's on the move. The bloodwork is inconclusive because there are no cancer markers.

"Some people don't get them even if they have the disease," he explains, adding that he's thrown out the blood test results because two different scans confirm the rapidly moving and multiplying malignant cells.

Regardless of fact, we seize on a germ of the idea that not having cancer indicators might be important, and it gives us a little something to grasp as positive. Not having the markers becomes even more significant because soon I'm on a modified macrobiotic diet and work like mad to eliminate toxins from my body.

The cancer is rated terminal, and I'm given six months to live. I might live two more years with chemotherapy and good luck, the doctor states:

"If you were a seventy-nine-year-old man, I'd send you home, observe you, and make you comfortable."

He tells me they can biopsy the largest tumor if we want further confirmation that the cells are malignant but says, based on his expertise, the cancerous lymph nodes assure him they are. He believes a biopsy would waste time, effort, and money. He then presents us with two options, both including chemotherapy. But he wants to run another diagnostic x-ray, and upon doing so, reinforces his assessment: I am sick with the deadliest stage of colon cancer and am in for the fight of my life!

When we ask about our planned Fourth of July trip to the Outer Banks, the doctor replies, "You need to more fully recover from surgery and grow stronger before you start therapy. Go to the beach, and have a good time. We'll begin chemo in August after you return home."

I can't suppress the thought that this might be my last vacation.

When David leaves for work the following morning, I call my friend Barbara Brinson to ask if she wants me to tell her about the oncologist's analysis or if she'd like to come over and hear the audio tape of the meeting.

She opts to come to our home and listen to his comments, so the two of us crawl onto the coverlet of my four-poster bed, place the tape recorder between us, hold hands, and cry as we listen to more than an hour of dialogue about my health. We remain silent except for the weeping . . . again, there are no words to voice our tumultuous emotions.

Barbara and I felt an instantaneous connection at our very first meeting. She was the visual arts teacher, and I taught theater arts at the local high school. We immediately recognized our kindred spirits and had been best friends for twenty-four years at the time of my diagnosis.

She is retired, so she has free time and promises to stand by me during my battle. The gift of herself and her time is definitely another God-Incidence. Barbara vows to be with me every step of the way and to help me carry the burden as I fight Cancer.

"I'll do it all with you!" she declares. Lighthearted but sincere, she proclaims she'll even shave her head in solidarity when I lose my hair due to the toxic medicines.

Unbeknownst to me, Barbara takes David aside to tell him to go to work and try not to worry. Her presence makes it possible for him to continue to earn a living with the understanding that I'm being safely tended to by her competent and compassionate hands. She assures him she'll give me the support I need when he's not physically available, and she is with me nearly every day for seven months.

Barbara is one of the countless earthly angels whose kindheartedness and interactions lift and encourage me; they help me grasp that even as I engage in battle with Cancer, I'm not trapped—I have the power to win this war!

David, too, has a best friend from work, Gary Ellison. I'm told later that Gary is a consistent source of encouragement for my husband during my recovery. My spouse had encouraged Gary when his wife survived breast cancer—now their roles are reversed.

"Try to stay positive," Gary advises David. "You'll get through the crisis as a team. Try to flow with the emotions rather than fight them. Take it one day at a time."

Through their unwavering friendships, Barbara and Gary bring us reassurance and exquisite care; without their loving support, the journey would have been far more difficult. We remain exceedingly thankful for the blessings they are in our lives.

Life Lesson #11: *Express gratitude; never hesitate to appreciate and thank individuals who positively affect your life.*

Barbara and I have surrounded each other with empathy in times of happiness and sorrow. I am an only child, and we could not be closer if we were sisters. She's an accomplished professional visual artist, an extraordinary educator, a brilliant scholar, and a loyal friend. Her heart's as big as the whole outdoors. A giver, caretaker, and peacemaker, she's mentored and inspired hundreds of students who adore her. Just knowing her has made me a better person.

Her spirit, compassion, quick thinking, and comic timing amaze me, as her brain computes and responds rapidly, a skill I envy, for I am dyslexic. Sometimes, it takes me a while to come up with a rejoinder, but not Barbara! She expresses herself magnificently and constantly impresses me with her witticisms, creativity, and vast knowledge.

Another manifestation of dyslexia is in my speech. David says I write from my brain and talk from my mouth—and my mouth often surprises us with its hilarious disconnect from the intellectual instrument!

Barbara's husband, Jim, is our great friend, and the four of us get together often, make memories, and laugh.

"You know something?" Barbara cheerfully confides one day as she accompanies me to one of my doctor's appointments. "There are very few people on this planet whom I love unconditionally, and you are one of them." My heart swells, for I feel the same way about her. Blessed with both David and Barbara, I am forever grateful.

We do not know it now, but my friend's proclamation of unconditional love foreshadows the most meaningful lesson I will learn on this journey.

Life Lesson #12: *Unconditional love is a most precious gift; acknowledging it is overwhelmingly sweet.*

Barbara, miserable after listening to my audio-taped diagnosis, feels she needs time alone. Although her intention for that bleak Thursday night was to take her mother to an art class, due to my devastating news, her husband accompanies her mom to the Artist Cooperative, locally referred to as *The Coop*, for a clay class.

Perceptive and intuitive, Barbara's quiet time prompts direction when she realizes a sudden, surprising compulsion to *"go to The Coop . . . go to The Coop . . . ."* Upon realizing it's vital for her to do so, she pulls herself together and drives to class.

"My best friend is dying of cancer, and I don't know what to do!" she exclaims as she bursts through the door, and nearly everyone mumbles "sorry" as twelve pairs of eyes look up at her and eleven pairs of eyes revert quickly back to their clay.

When they hear the word *cancer*, many people do not know what to do or say. In the past, my response has been similar. Now, because of my experience with the disease, I offer hope, positive thoughts, and prayers for the healing of those who must deal with deadly personal invasions. (*Well-meaning friends sometimes share dreadful cancer stories that are devastating for the diagnosed to hear. I urge everyone reading this to understand that it's imperative to think before you speak and that stepping into the role of cancer warrior is best served through supportive compassion.*)

As Barbara crosses the classroom, she reiterates, "Jimmi-Ann's dying of cancer, and there's nothing I can do . . ."

"Oh, this is great news! Do I have a story to tell you!" exclaims the twelfth artist. She surprises Barbara when she jumps out of her chair and declares: "My mother had Stage 4 breast cancer, and she's alive and well—three years later! I can help your friend!"

This woman, Renée Brigman, emanates such excitement, energy, and sincerity that my friend listens in awe, astonished. And within a few minutes, Barbara's world evolves from devastating sadness to enthusiastic hope.

Renée's words (excerpt from **The Cancer Cookbook**): "In January of 2003, my mom, Emilie, was diagnosed with Stage IV metastatic breast cancer. It had grown into her lung and into her spine. The prognosis was horrific; Mother had very little time left, and conventional chemotherapy offered very little hope. We decided to do chemo, but it looked like the herbal world offered more.

Since Emilie's mother, my grandmother, and several of her sisters had also been diagnosed with breast cancer, the real possibility existed that it was only a matter of time until my three sisters and I would be faced with the same diagnosis. We decided that if the cancer wasn't genetic, then it was most likely environmentally triggered. The more we learned about the links between food and breast cancer, the more terrified we became. Then, we discovered Roxanne Koteles and **The Cancer Cookbook**. If food was killing people, we wondered: Could food save them, too?

After consulting with Roxanne, we recognized her commitment to everyone being healthy and whole. Instantly, she became part of our team to make Mom well. She explained her realistic approach to changing our way of eating and, thus our way of life. Emilie's life became family first and food second. Coming from an Italian heritage, food—really good, tasty food—was a huge part of our daily lives. And to give it all up seemed impossible.

But with Roxanne as our guide, we did it! Although my mother attacked the cancer with traditional chemotherapy, she's certain that the herbs, and especially the food plan, were instrumental to her recovery. Her tumor measured 40 x 50 mm and the tumor markers registered at 79 in January 2003. By March of 2004, the tumor did not register enough to measure and by May of that year, the cancer markers were down to 9.8. And Emilie is so proud of her svelte new figure!"[1]

Hearing Emilie's story and the passion with which Renée conveys it, Barbara shifts from hopelessness to optimism.

Life Lesson #13: *Hopelessness is not a strategy; positivity is power.*

Renée supplies the necessary contact information, and my friend heads home to call Roxanne, whose first available consultation appointment isn't until Wednesday. Disappointed at having to wait, Barbara knows she has no choice and calls me to tell me about her plan.

At first, I'm tentative about rushing off to see someone I know little about. But Barbara's emotional shift from despair to hope becomes contagious, and I resolve to go, realizing I'll try just about anything to survive. I've barely hung up the telephone when it rings again—it's Barb, and she's excited:

"*Every* client Roxanne is scheduled to see on Friday has canceled their appointments, so she can see us tomorrow!"

Call it serendipity or phenomenon; I decide to follow the path that's opening to me. Two God-Incidences within a few hours! A seed for a miracle has just been planted, and we have no idea how much one phone call will change all of our lives.

Life Lesson #14: *Trust that the unexpected can lead to amazing possibilities.*

SCENE 4

Radical Changes in My Wisdom Regarding Food:
Setting the Stage for Successfully Conquering the Disease

"I'm going to live! Food is the key!
Right-food is an essential remedy!"
~ JIMMI-ANN

David and Barbara, always my greatest fans, are now my greatest guardians. Barbara opens the door that leads us to an incredible woman, Roxanne Koteles, who becomes our food coach, and her program becomes my lifeline. I adhere steadfastly to *FoodWisdomRx*™, Roxanne's modified macrobiotic food plan, and the results are astonishing.[2] I had been given several "kicks in the backside" through my various health problems, and although I understood that I should be treating my body as a temple, it is easiest to do nothing. So now the temple is crumbling.

My immune system has been a wreck for at least a decade; my general practitioner consistently encouraged me to get it in shape. I neglected to take care of myself by doing the work necessary to achieve wellness. *The* cancer diagnosis becomes a slap up the side of my head, and it's high time I pay attention!

ACT 1 SCENE 4

Late Friday morning, Barbara drives us to Arden, North Carolina, just outside Asheville, to meet with Roxanne at her home. We giggle and laugh on the two-hour drive up the mountain, speculating about who and what we'll find. Like "Lucy and Ethel," we are routinely cavorting cohorts in outrageous episodes—here we are, off on another escapade, a road trip to see a complete stranger to *learn how to eat!*

Who is this woman we're going to meet?

Is she as good as Renée has led Barbara to believe?

Will she be a lunatic?

Might she be a leftover hippie with long, gray, stringy hair entwined with flowers and wearing love beads?

Will she be chanting with incense burning in ashtrays—or something worse?

We hold hands, take deep breaths, and ring the doorbell.

A petite, energetic fireball opens the door—and her heart—to us as we enter the world of *FoodWisdomRx*™. A whirlwind of information and calculation, Roxanne takes one look at me and declares, "I can definitely help you!"

She grabs my hand, pulls me to her back deck, and says: "I have to take *before* pictures." Then she snaps photographs of my face and feet!

Barbara and I eyeball each other the whole time.

Feet pictures!

Feet pictures?

Lord have mercy—what have we gotten ourselves into?

"I'm not worried about you," Roxanne enthuses, "we'll clear you up in no time!"

Is she for real?

She proceeds to "read" my face and feet and explains later that she studied oriental medicine, a practice that's been around since ancient times.

It's all very, very strange to us.

An acclaimed cook who left the Ritz-Carlton in San Francisco to help people get well through proper diet, she studied macrobiotic cooking, diagnosis healing, philosophy, and shiatsu at the Kushi Institute, the world's leading center for macrobiotic education.

At the time, I didn't realize she was using visual diagnostic techniques to evaluate my health.

Today, I describe Roxanne as vital, healthy, and energetic, with exceptional nutritional and medical knowledge, but at the time, we watch, wonder, and worry.

"In my program, you'll learn how to use powerful healing foods and energy currents in the body to bring about extraordinary changes in your health and well-being," she informs me.

These concepts are foreign, peculiar, weird—even bizarre.

I'm not convinced.

Given that I often battled weight issues, I believe I've heard and tried it all before. I think I know just about all there is to know about diet, but I'm about to discern just how little I understand about nutrition.

She assesses me as having high blood pressure and a proclivity for diabetes, heart failure, arthritis, cancer, and depression.

Roxanne does this just by looking at my mug and my tootsies?

Skeptical, I figure anyone with weight issues would have these problems. Cancer is pretty darn depressing, and she knew about the malignancy before she opened the door and invited us inside.

The uneasiness about what she is offering increases.

Roxanne finishes my preliminary evaluation, turns to Barbara, and says: "I'm more concerned about you than Jimmi-Ann. She's no problem; we'll fix her up in no time! I'm going to put you guys on the family plan—it's less expensive that way, and the two of you are going to do this together!"

Our jaws drop as the red-headed tornado then photographs and tags Barbara!

ACT 1 SCENE 4

Roxanne commences to list six issues that Barbara has with her health.

We gasp again, this time in astonishment!

Earlier in the week, my friend had seen her doctor for the results of medical tests he'd run. Our new coach now tells Barbara *exactly* what her physician had revealed. And she does this by looking at her face and feet?

Flabbergasting.

Another God-Incidence!

We have absolute proof that we're in the right place—instant verification that we're doing exactly what we are supposed to do!

Roxanne sits us down in her living room and begins to explain her food plan. We take notes quickly, but fortunately, she audio tapes the session for us, talking for over an hour as we try fruitlessly to absorb everything she's saying.

I look across the room at Barbara, and she appears as gob-smacked as I feel. Nevertheless, she gives me a weak smile, and we both turn our attention back to the information. There's *sooooo* much to internalize.

Impressed, I grab this lifeline and hold on for dear life!

This program presents real hope for conquering the disease!

With amusement, Roxanne recalls that we both looked like deer caught in headlights and took turns crying like crazy women during the consultation. She realized she had two *characters* on her hands and felt a connection with us that would become more than that of a food coach to her clients.

The main idea of *FoodWisdomRx*™ is to view food from an entirely new perspective. Roxanne leads the way for us to connect with quality foods like those we consumed in childhood before additives and genetically modified organisms (GMOs) became standard.

We ask questions.

She clearly explains how processed and preserved foods are killing us.

She introduces us to organics and explains why it's important to eat foods with names we can't even pronounce.

We ask questions.

Roxanne enlightens us about the energy in food and how it affects our bodies.

We ask questions.

She discusses the importance of balance in all aspects of life: mind, body, spirit, *and* nutrition.

We have even more questions.

She lectures, demonstrates, and explains, telling us which foods I should eliminate from my diet to stop feeding *the* cancer.

We learn that an effective way to fight it is to starve malignant cells by not supplying them with the foods they require to multiply and spread.

We listen.

We learn.

My intuition, my God-Voice, assures me that the answer to our prayers is being revealed.

We are being shown the way!

I'm going to put this plan into action!

Life Lesson #15: *Listen to your intuition, your God-Voice, and take action accordingly.*

The principal items to be eliminated from our diets include *sugar, dairy, meat, caffeine,* and *gluten.*

Sugar: Every cell in our body uses glucose as its primary food source; however, cancer cells absorb sugar very quickly. Eliminating sugar and simple carbohydrates from a diet helps to slow the growth of the cells.

Dairy products: Casein in dairy is a culprit that stimulates tumor cell growth, and dairy products also create mucus in the body, making it more susceptible to disease.

Meat: Animal protein is fatty and difficult to digest, compromising the body when cancer is present as fat feeds the rapidly multiplying cells.

Caffeine: Caffeine has a high acid content; if the body's PH balance is acidic, this supports the rapid growth of the disease. Even with decaffeination, we ingest carcinogenic chemicals that rinse away coffee's caffeine and residual pesticides. An exception is a Swiss-washed decaffeination, which still contributes some acid to your PH balance.

These four foods encourage the rapid growth of malignant cells.

Gluten: We're also told to eliminate gluten since it damages the body because it gums up the plumbing. Roxanne encourages a gluten-free lifestyle for every client.

Barbara is to adhere to the same plan, for it will also address her health issues.

The program is an elimination diet that works to remove toxins and candida, a fungal infection caused by yeast. Most people have yeast overgrowth because of their food choices and from taking antibiotics.

Roxanne recommends quality products, vitamins, supplements, probiotics, and gut solutions as critical additions to *FoodWisdomRx*™. This new way of eating also produces rapid weight loss, and we're thrilled with that aspect of the plan!

Life Lesson #16: *Just because something is unusual or beyond your experience, give it a chance; it might be exactly what you need.*

Six years earlier, when my doctor diagnosed me as being a celiac, I stopped eating wheat and felt better for it. The gastroenterologist observed that the damage to my small intestine had been repaired by cutting wheat from my diet, my irritable bowel syndrome (IBS) had disappeared, and the inflammation in my joints was greatly lessened.

Looking back, I realize that celiac disease was another God-Incidence preparing me to adapt to this new food plan more easily. Celiac disease is an autoimmune disorder of the small intestine; symptoms often include chronic diarrhea and exhaustion.

Caused by a reaction to gluten found in wheat, exposure to gluten causes an inflammatory reaction inside the bowel tissue that leads to a reduction of the villi. Villi are tiny thread-like projections that line the small intestine and distribute nutrients throughout the entire body. The villi are responsible for nutrient absorption, so their destruction hampers the assimilation of nutrients. A lifelong gluten-free diet allowing the intestinal lining and the villi to recover is the only known treatment for celiac disease. [3]

In general, when I stopped eating gluten in 1999, gluten-free items tasted like sawdust or cardboard. Since then, there have been significant advances in the taste and texture of these products. However, an aggravating thing about living a gluten-free existence is the way it is concealed under other names in many products as a flavor enhancer.

I'd eliminated gluten six years earlier.

I can do this!

I can follow the modified macrobiotic diet!

I can do the *FoodWisdom* plan!

Hippocrates, the father of modern medicine, introduced the term *macrobiotics* to describe people who are healthy and long-lived.[4] He wrote about the importance of balance in mind, body, and spirit. He believed that exercise and a diet of fresh, seasonal foods resulted in a long and healthy life.

A traditional macrobiotic diet involves removing gluten from the diet but eating good grains as the primary food source, supplemented with beans and vegetables. Macrobiotic eating avoids the use of highly processed or refined foods.

Roxanne's culinary expertise allowed her to devise a program that is tasty rather than bland. It doesn't employ nearly as many grains as the original diet. Also, she allows fish, permits chicken on a rotating basis, and says shellfish is okay once in a while. Her program is designed to keep the body, tissues, and organs moist rather than drying them out as a traditional macrobiotic regimen often does.

We are to adopt an organic lifestyle with vegetables, proteins, and gluten-free grains as staples of her plan. Some berries and fruits are allowed.

It's all about balance and portions.

Our new guru gives us a daily menu to follow unwaveringly for the first month. It looks doable.

Barbara is sending out non-verbal messages that scream: *Help! Help! I can't do this! What have we gotten ourselves into?*

However, she soon dissolves into laughter because she says I became as delighted as a small child with a treat when I discover that we're allowed half a banana at lunchtime during the third week of the elimination diet—and I don't particularly like bananas!

Although we're both shell-shocked, Barbara is stunned and filled with admiration that I so quickly and emphatically get on board with the program. I'm ecstatic with the hope this plan has ignited.

Hope—what a beautiful concept!

There's *action* I can take to change my circumstances!

Cancer becomes a beatable foe!

Of course, I'm ecstatic! Barbara becomes my North Star, guiding me to a place where I can begin to feel safe once again. We don't realize we're setting the stage for even more Miracles.

Life Lesson #17: *Miracles come in many different guises; pay attention and accept them with loving gratitude.*

Roxanne provides a grocery list and, with our heads spinning, shows us the door. Waving with encouragement, she sends us to the nearest organic supermarket to make purchases for our new lifestyle. She provides a phone number to call if and when we have questions or need her assistance.

We crawl back into the car, look at each other, and take a deep breath . . .

What the hell just happened?

SCENE 5

Extraordinary Misadventure!
Upon Reflection: Grocery Store Calamity Becomes Comedic Episode!

"Barbara, are you sure this is an adventure?"
~ JIMMI-ANN

Chaotically overwhelmed with besieged brains and rebellious bodies, we're dog-tired and practically cross-eyed from the consultation! I'm a week off major surgery—frazzled and beyond exhaustion.

"Did you understand all of that?" I ask Barbara.

"No . . ."

"Me neither . . . but I'm going to do it. *I feel like I'm supposed to do it.*"

"Well, I'm doing it too!"

"Do you feel like going to get groceries?"

"No. But I'm going anyway." With that, she puts her Highlander into reverse, and off we head to the organic market.

Years ago, my family doctor persuaded me to go organic because of my weakened immune system. After trying it for two weeks, I complained, "It's too expensive. It's not worth it."

After just one session with Roxanne, I understand how erroneous that statement had been. I have suffered for years with IBS, adrenal fatigue, exhaustion, aching joints, dermatographia, skin tags, and dry skin. I learned that all of these are symptoms that have to do with wrong-eating. Relatively quickly, with right-eating, every single one of these issues disappears.

Organic eating is the foundation of my new lifestyle plan.

Certifiably organic foods must also be free of artificial additives and processed with as few non-natural conditions as possible. Chemical ripening, food irradiation, and genetically modified ingredients are generally not permitted. The use of growth hormones and antibiotics are not allowed in organics.

Today's over-processed foods lack vital nutrients, while GMOs, antibiotics, hormones, pesticides, chemical cleansing agents, and other contaminants are routinely found in conventional foods. Bisphenol-A (BPAs, an industrial chemical used in plastics manufacturing and added to many commercial products, including food containers, baby bottles, plastic water bottles, and hygiene products) is another contaminant that compromises our health.

Eating organic foods is much less expensive in the long run than doctors' medications, surgeries, and other treatments that may result from a conventional diet. I now prefer the produce department of an organic supermarket to a drug store.

Life Lesson #18: *Clean, organic foods are a pathway to wellness.*

Barbara and I are notorious for getting lost because we inevitably become giddy from our conversations. Fortunately, we're too worn out to talk as we drive straight to the grocery.

In 2005, going organic was far from mainstream. We learn from Roxanne that organic food stores are dedicated to marketing the freshest and healthiest foods available. These stores do not allow artificial flavors, colors, preservatives, and hydrogenated oils. Plus, natural food stores support the local economy and organic farms. Just what our food coach ordered! In fact, she sends clients to the Asheville store, which partners with *FoodWisdomRx*™ and guarantees to help buyers with their purchases.

ACT 1 SCENE 5

As Barb pulls into the parking lot, I confess I'm too exhausted to shop and that my incision is throbbing. As miserable as I am, Barbara is nevertheless determined to continue today's unfolding drama.

"That's OK. I'll do it for both of us," she announces, grinning. "You sit out here at a table, put your feet up, and rest!"

"I'm shattered! Aren't you too worn out to do this today?"

"No. I'm fine," Barbara replies as she peruses the long, long, long grocery list, "This shouldn't be too bad . . . besides, we don't want to drive back up here tomorrow, do we?"

Even though she's not fooling me by denying her fatigue, I acquiesce. But I'm too weary to protest. I permit my dear friend to enter the *organic cosmos* alone! Barbara Brinson becomes an extraordinary trailblazer! She's going way beyond the call of duty!

I am ashamed of my desertion, but I don't let that stop me from releasing a deep sigh, putting my feet up, and focusing wholeheartedly on breathing and relaxing . . .

I fall into a deep, deep sleep.

I wake up over an hour later and realize my best friend is missing in action!

Guilt kicks in, followed immediately by an epiphany! One of our problems is the lack of fuel!

FOOD! Food is fuel!

No wonder we're worn out!

We haven't eaten since breakfast, and it's nearly dinnertime!

We. Require. Fuel.

Somehow, I summon enough energy to stand up and wobble into the store.

I discover Barbara with two buggies filled to the brim, almost ready to checkout. Her ever-present charisma has obviously charmed the store manager who's graciously helping her.

She looks dreadful! Then I realize that I mirror her appallingly terrible demeanor. We both look unhinged, with scraggly hair, pallid complexions, rumbling bellies, and wild, vacant looks in our eyes. Mercifully, we aren't drooling—yet.

Her personal shopper continues to gather more items and then gallantly pushes my buggy to the cash register as I attempt to help Barbara move hers.

Fortunately, we're too pooped to pass out when our bills are totaled. Each receipt is well over three hundred dollars—and that's in 2005! Included are vitamins and supplements that Roxanne deems essential, lots of fresh vegetables, and plenty of items to restock our pantries after we clean out the "un-eatables" at home.

Mind you, many purchases are part of a starter kit, and there are items we won't have to purchase again soon because they have a super long shelf life. When we run out of an item, we can replace it. But happily, everything won't run out all at once.

Barbara manages to load the SUV with all our bags. I can't help her because I'm forbidden to lift anything that weighs more than five pounds due to my surgery. Besides, we certainly don't want my insides spilling out all over the place!

I persuade her to let me return the carts to the store and stagger back to the car while holding tight to the elastic band encircling my middle.

Ravenous, we dive into the paper bags to find something to vanquish our hunger!

Somewhat fortified by inhaling organic rice chips and almond butter, Barbara's restored enough to relate what happened in the store while I snoozed outside . . .

She sees a young staff member and requests assistance:

"Hey there! I sure will be grateful if you can help me with this—I just don't know where to start!" She gives him the very long list—he grudgingly lends a hand, sighing and grunting repeatedly while retrieving various items.

Exasperated, she finally says, "Hon, if you don't want to help me, you don't have to!"

He disappears like smoke in the wind . . .

Barbara is stunned.

At the point of meltdown, hopelessly adrift in a strange organic universe, she considers a tantrum. She contemplates throwing herself on the floor, pounding her fists, and kicking her feet. Fortunately, she's too tired, too responsible, and, as she proclaims, too old, though it is very tempting.

Enter the Big Boss: to the rescue!

Spying a wilted woman with two half-full grocery carts—clearly frustrated and about to collapse—the store manager salvages Barbara's misadventure! And not a moment too soon, as her brainwaves are not fully functioning. She has no idea what to do. He rescues her with kindness as he listens to her calamitous account. He expresses disappointment in the attitude of his employee and compassionately assists her with her list.

He recognizes our purchases as Roxanne's *Critical Care Level Supply Kit* and explains to Barbara the benefits of kombu, miso, kuzu, and wakame. He affirms Roxanne's choice of vitamins and supplements and helps conclude the overwhelming and exhaustive adventure positively, although it is still costly.

What is money when life hangs in the balance?

While the price tag is high, we *know* we're on the path to healing!

We find out later that the staff was reminded that Roxanne's clients are a top priority and should be treated as important and with respect. The one churlish stock boy who disregarded those instructions and later became belligerent with his superior is now gone. Her new clients are guaranteed a better experience thanks to poor Barbara's distress.

Life Lesson #19: *Showing compassion is a matter of choice; becoming aware of the feelings of others helps us make kindhearted choices.*

My husband, David, greets two hollow-eyed, bedraggled females upon our return home. "Lucy and Ethel" collapse into the living room.

Sizing up the situation immediately, he tells us to relax as he delivers my purchases to the kitchen. I request that he only put away things needing refrigeration because I have to get acquainted with the other items.

Eventually, Barbara and I look at each other, haul ourselves up, and lurch toward the kitchen.

David, recognizing the climate, escapes as quickly as possible!

Still starving, we decide to try a greens drink, which is to become part of our daily menu to give us energy. Our depleted *get-up-and-go* desperately needs rescuing!

Green foods boost the immune system because they contain chlorella, algae, seaweed, and powerful phytonutrients.[5] Phytonutrients are natural chemicals in food that cleanse the body and blood to help it work efficiently. They help prevent oxidation by providing antioxidants such as vitamins C, E, and beta-carotene.

Oxidation is believed to encourage diseases like cancer, diabetes, and neurodegenerative disorders; oxidative stress can damage cells and promote aging.

Green foods enhance immunity and protect against illness as they assist digestion, reduce inflammation, and help prevent cancer. Containing alkaline-forming minerals, these greens help prevent the body from becoming acidic. An acidic environment encourages diseases like cancer, heart disease, arthritis, and digestive and respiratory tract disorders.

Acting bravely, if not convincingly, I pull out the container of greens concentrate and the blender. We measure the powder and add water, aloe vera juice, wild cherry concentrate, a quarter cup of blueberries, and some other mysterious natural ingredients. After blending, I pour the mixture into two glasses.

ACT 1 SCENE 5

Our eyes and noses automatically rebel.

We peer at the opaque brew, look at each other, and simultaneously say, "It's *greeeeeeeen* . . ."

It *is green.*

Really green . . .

Unappetizing.

Neither of us dare taste it.

I take a deep breath, grin at my collaborator, and exclaim: "Let's see if Davy likes it!"

We limp into the study where he is reading, smile sweetly, and I coo, "Does this look good to you?"

I hold out the goblet of green slime for him to inspect. He closes his book, grins, and sighs. "You want *me* to taste it?" our two heads bobble as he takes a gulp and manages to keep it down.

"It's not too bad," he grimaces.

My sweetheart has now become my food taster!

Life Lesson #20: *If you have an incredible partner, express your appreciation frequently!*

We thank him profusely and, in view of the fact that he didn't croak, go out on the porch to drink. We figure if we should hurl it will be over the railing instead of making more of a mess for David to clean up. Housework by two walking disasters is not an option—we're having enough difficulty just lifting our glasses because we're so depleted!

We toast to good health, hold our noses, and swallow.

It's barely palatable, but we manage to get it down and determine that disguising the green sludge in clay mugs the next time will help ingestion.

Amazingly, within a week, we begin to look forward to *greens drink time* because our food preferences have radically changed, and we now consider this beverage a delicious indulgence!

Meanwhile, eliminating sugar and simple carbohydrates frees our taste buds to experience authentic flavors and textures. As cravings disappear, we begin to anticipate little "mouth-watering parties" at every meal!

Life Lesson #21: *Don't be afraid to try new things; you might just be pleased and surprised at the outcome.*

SCENE 6

A New Life in the Kitchen:
Vegetables–Southern Manner of Preparation Strictly Prohibited!

> "Let's get some good ole appetizers
> just to get things started!
>
> Sweetie, would you bring me coconut shrimp
> with mango dressing, chicken and dumplings,
> a double cheeseburger with bacon, sweet
> barbeque—can't eat barbeque without
> coleslaw . . . a loaded baked potato,
> and some banana puddin'?
>
> Oooh, don't forget hot apple cobbler
> with ice cream!
>
> Now, David, it's your turn—order your favorites."
> ~ JIMMI-ANN

We begin implementing one element of the *FoodWisdomRx* program immediately—morning teas. Roxanne had prepared the beverages for us at her home and advised us to drink them on Saturday and Sunday before we start her program on Monday. We will make these two Japanese drinks from scratch each morning to start our day because they are fundamental to alkalizing our bodily systems.

My body chemistry has been acidic long enough for cancer cells to grow and rapidly develop. Now, the question is whether I'll be able to stop and reverse the process by employing prayer, foods, traditional medicine, supplements, and a positive attitude.

Can I survive a modified macrobiotic lifestyle?

Digestive enzymes are vital to a healthy body and occur naturally in some plants and fruit. They are also heat-sensitive. *FoodWisdomRx* allows cooked vegetables, but not those cooked at high temperatures. Vegetables cooked above 118 degrees Fahrenheit are not used in macrobiotics because their aid to digestion becomes deactivated.

Freshly made vegetable juice offers live enzymes that are easily absorbed and reach cellular levels quickly to encourage the growth of healthy cells. Drinking fresh juice and eating raw vegetables several times a day is fundamental.

Roxanne encourages fish consumption because it's high in Omega 3s and easily absorbed into the body. Chicken is allowed on a rotating basis for variety, although it is difficult to digest. Protein is essential for extra energy, natural minerals, and vitamins.

I wonder if we can *improve our health by including this holistic approach to healing*. I hope so because I firmly believe that additional lifestyle changes will help me conquer Cancer.

My "new life" is to begin that first Monday, so I pig out one final time on Saturday and Sunday. During those two days, I consume a steak, baked potato, potato chips, a BLT, and a couple of hamburgers—minus the bread—and ice cream. I devour Hershey's Kisses. I have no idea how I'll enjoy life without this fodder. I'd pretty much given up soft drinks but guzzle a couple before Monday morning. My typical pre-diet thinking is that I need one last binge before depriving myself of the foods I enjoy—foods that comfort me.

Shock! Surprise! Revelation!

Eating the right foods in the correct manner eliminates cravings and creates cuisine connoisseurs!

After a few weeks of competent eating, Barbara and I discover that taking comfort from heavy foods is a false notion. We become food snobs, no longer craving or even wanting the very fare that had been killing us!

David and I enjoy a beautiful, well-equipped kitchen but rarely use it on weekdays because we traverse "restaurant row" on our way home from work. After a long day of energetic teaching, it's much easier to dine out. Restaurants must now be avoided; I eventually understand how to manipulate their menus and remain on the program. However, I prepare nearly every meal I eat over the next year.

My spouse proves himself to be a blessing again by going on the plan with me, so I don't have to prepare separate meals for him. This man, who ate antacids like candy for years, quickly neutralizes his stomach acid and is now off the tablets! By following this new lifestyle plan, David drops weight, and his health shows improvement—in three days both of his blood pressure numbers decrease by twenty points and have since remained in the normal range.

Roxanne explains that a person with overall good health can stray from her program a couple of times a week and stay healthy. David is happy with the program as he *interprets* her statement to mean that an occasional slice of cake or a cheap gas station hotdog isn't going to wreck his constitution!

It's all about choices.

Life Lesson #22: *It is true that we are what we eat! We may use food to improve our health or to hurt our bodies.*

Following the plan's thirty-day menu is much easier because Barbara and I are doing it together. Although we prepare food in our separate households, we have each other for support. It was brilliant to put both of us on the program because it makes us hold each other responsible for adhering to it and makes staying on it more pleasurable.

Barbara makes astonishing, rapid progress concerning her medical issues—all six are addressed and quickly improve with nutrition.

I always enjoyed eating vegetables, but I grew up in the South, where massacring them is tradition. Boiled, fried, or fricasseed to a limp, pale, pastel color, they were inevitably prepared with real butter, fatback, bacon, or ham. Our new way of preparing plants calls for very little cooking time, resulting in the retention of nutrients, their vibrant color, and crispness. They taste yummy, as do the new grains I introduce to my palate.

I discover additional gluten-free products that taste good on Roxanne's plan. She provides incredible recipes that elevate diet to gourmet.

We love it!

Here's a side note about God's wisdom: I had eliminated all wheat and grains from my diet except rice, oats, and corn for six years. Now I'm introduced to good-tasting gluten-free items, and I feel as if I'm being rewarded with something I previously had to do without! Imagine that—I feel *rewarded* by what I eat on her program!

A coincidence?

I think not!

A God-Incidence to help ensure my success!

Eating vegetables first thing in the morning is uncharted territory, but I've come to appreciate the taste and energy they give me early in the day. Very basically, the plan has three classifications of vegetables, and we should eat some of them at every meal. While the *FoodWisdomRx* regimen is much more complicated, these vegetables are essentially what we consume as we rotate proteins.

Natural food tastes great when we don't smother it with sauces and gravies. Surprised to learn that working with food can be a pleasure, I discover there's nothing like the taste of authentic flavors!

Everything's going well our first few days on the program, but I panic when I notice we're supposed to have tofu the next morning.

TOFU?

Yikes!

Yuck! Yuck! Yuck!

Coagulated soybean curd!

YUCK!

My face automatically screws up at the thought of having to cook the gelatinous substance.

It has the gross factor.

It stops me cold!

Immediately on the phone with Barbara, I announce that I'm coming to her house for breakfast tomorrow!

My friend has no problem with the stuff. In fact, during her salad days, she grew soybeans and made her own tofu.

A tofu expert has been provided!

Coincidence?

Not!

Bright and early the next day, she chops and sautés a small onion in a minute amount of toasted sesame oil as I stand by observing. Next, she opens the dreaded tofu, pours off the water, and lays it on a chopping block.

"I'm just going to prepare half of it," she says as she slides a knife through the gunk.

"Lord have mercy," my stomach quivers.

"Here, can you please put the rest into a baggie?"

"Ew, that means I have to touch the glob...." I mumble under my breath.

"Just do it!"

"Yikes!" I'm surprised when I manage to handle it without gagging.

"It's really good," Barbara remarks.

"Yeah, just like the greens drink, I'm sure..."

"You'll be surprised," she adds, "just like the greens drink, it grows on you."

"*Yeah, like mildew,*" I softly complain.

She drops the small cubes into the pan with the onion and oil.

"I can tell I'm *really* going to like it," I sarcastically mumble.

Surprisingly, the aroma of the onion and oil smells heavenly as the tofu begins to brown. It looks beautiful, too, just like hash browns—I've certainly put away plenty of those in my day!

Barbara throws in a handful of chopped kale, carrots, and mushrooms, transfers it to a small pot, then adds water and a half cup of organic marinara sauce. She continues to heat it until the soup simmers; it smells wonderful . . .

We grab a cup of Kukicha Twig Tea and a bowl of soup, then head for the porch.

Twig tea, Kukicha, is made from the stems, stalks, and twigs of the green tea plant. Highly beneficial, it's loaded with antioxidants and very low in caffeine. Effective in neutralizing the body's acid levels and rich in natural tannins, it often evokes a feeling of well-being.

We sit, silently rocking, our senses elevated by this little piece of paradise created by the Brinsons in their beautifully landscaped, wooded hideaway, absorbing the sights, sounds, and smells, thrilled to be in this delightful garden of Eden.

Eventually, I have to face the tofu, so I revert to my "you-go-first" mode again.

"Mmmmm," is all Barbara says after taking a bite.

I take a deep breath, pick up my spoon, exhale, and put it down. "I don't think I can do this!"

"Drink your tea. I'll eat yours," Barbara twinkles.

She knows me so very well . . .

I grab the spoon and take a small portion.

Surprise!

It isn't so bad!

The more I consume, the better it tastes.

ACT 1 SCENE 6

We both go back for seconds!

We've now become adept in the kitchen. Barbara doesn't enjoy cooking, but I find myself inspired by the activity as I like to create dishes to meet Roxie's high standards.

I dislike washing up a disassembled, dirty kitchen after I've enjoyed a meal, but Roxanne teaches us that professionals clean as they go. Following that advice makes life much easier.

Roxanne and her sister Rosie, also a cooking specialist, have both given us cooking tutorials. As visual and performing artists, it's an eye-opening experience to work with trained professionals who see food as their art form. Chopping, slicing, dicing, and sautéing all require specific skills, just like sculpture, painting, acting, and mime.

Who would have thought?

As for the tofu?

We have become friends.

I'm no longer afraid of it and now know many delicious ways to prepare it.

Eventually, we cut back on soy products as the variety and availability of other food resources grew significantly.

However, I'll never forget my first tofu experience—a magnificent morning rewarded with a delightful, treasured memory: indulgence on Barbara's porch in the midst of a soft summer breeze, blossoms, butterflies, and bumblebees.

ACT II

POSSIBILITIES MULTIPLY AS BELIEF IN MIRACLES GROW

SCENE 1

Optimism Required:
Positive Thinking is Essential for Opening Doors to Miracles

"Oh, my goodness! Somehow, it's all about love.
Absolutely everything evolves from love!"
~ JIMMI-ANN

As my journey progresses, I come to believe that cancer is a disease of the mind, body, *and* soul. I firmly believe that inadequate nourishment of any of these components results in *dis*-ease.

A positive attitude and persevering spirit help *the* cancer Warrior become a survivor, and survivors must learn to temper negative emotions.

Anger, Guilt, Blame, Fear, and Resentment produce excessive cortisol hormones, resulting in bodily stress. Too much cortisol due to Anxiety and Worry leads to adrenal fatigue and places our bodies in an acidic environment. Remember, an acidic PH imbalance helps fuel malignant cells.

On June 25, 2005, one month out of surgery and forty-three days from the colonoscopy, the Warrior perseveres! *My gut feeling since the initial shock remains the same: I will heal!*

Following through with my oncologist's suggestion to go ahead and travel, we head for the Outer Banks.

I take my organic foodstuffs and am able to get plenty of freshly caught fish at the beach—and the two servings of shellfish my program allows. I stick to the requirements and discover that it only takes a smile, a simple explanation, or a polite request, and restaurants are happy to let me bring my own food—or even cook for me using my organic ingredients. It warms my heart because many folks go out of their way to be helpful!

Life Lesson #23: *Don't be afraid to advocate for yourself; most people will be happy to help if you are sincere and grateful.*

We've spent many vacations on the Outer Banks, and our first stop is picturesque Roanoke Island. It is there that I performed in America's oldest-running outdoor drama, *The Lost Colony*, in Manteo for six seasons; I acted in their touring show for three. I've cultivated roots in this coastal town as my home away from home because I find its rich history, welcoming community, and charm irresistible.

After a brief respite in Manteo and a visit with friends, we travel a bit further down the coast and experience a contemplative Fourth of July on Ocracoke Island, a small but lovely fishing village. It's a soothing experience—the warmhearted, friendly locals, the beauty, the relaxing atmosphere, and the 'magic' of the little town are a comfort to our raging emotions.

As we check out of the Bluff Shoal Motel, where we traditionally stay, the innkeeper asks if we'd like to go ahead and reserve our room for the following year. We always book a year in advance because the popular little inn fills up rapidly for the holiday week.

My heart nearly falls out of my body! *I won't be here! Next year, I won't be on the planet!*

"Of course we do!" David replies instantly. "We wouldn't miss it for the world!"

He knows exactly what to say to lift my spirit and feed my soul.

"You won't believe this, but the whole motel is available next Fourth of July," we're informed. "No one has booked yet for vacation."

"Reserve the whole thing!" David decrees excitedly. "All seven rooms! We'll bring the kids and grandkids up here for the Fourth and celebrate your recovery!"

I *knew* then that I'd be back the following year.

Might this be another God-Incidence?

Definitely.

Life Lesson #24: *Positive thinking is essential in every aspect of our lives and will open doors to miracles if we remain optimistic.*

David and I said for ages that we wanted to bring the extended family to the island; it took a cancer diagnosis for us to make it happen. Don't put off making precious memories; the best time for memories is right now!

The following July 4, 2006, three of our children, their spouses (minus one son-in-law who could not take vacation time), nine grandchildren, and one significant other joined us to celebrate my glorious, renewed health and America's birthday on Ocracoke.

"Pa-pa," says seven-year-old Claude Austin as he looks up at his grandfather after an adventurous morning exploring the maritime forest alongside the sound, "This is the best vacation of my *entire* life!"

It is . . . it is . . . oh, it definitely is!

Life Lesson #25: *Stop putting off things you want to do; life is to enjoy now—this very day!*

From my journal: *On July 8, 2006, I will go for another CT scan. I've been eating organic foods to live for three weeks. If the tumors appear smaller than they were on the first test, we'll just have to watch them. If they no longer exist, it will be the miracle I'm determined to obtain!*

Calm and peaceful during the scan, I focus on it being smaller or not there at all. I believe it will be diminished—or, better yet, completely vanished!

Not really.

My words are powerful, but my thoughts are not.

I'm not yet ready to *truly* believe.

As the oncologist surmised, I have Stage 4 cancer—the last, most terrible phase.

Stages 1 to 4 catalog how much *the* cancer has spread. The measurement is based on the size of a tumor, how deeply it's rooted, if it's spread to other organs, and how many lymph nodes are infected.

The classification at diagnosis is the best way to predict survival, and therapies are adjusted according to the depth of the invasion. I am all the way out there at the deadliest level. It actually helps me to pretend there are Stages 5, 6, and 7.

As we make arrangements to begin chemotherapy, my spirit continues to be strong, but oh, what a burden we carry.

Devastated once again, David and I drive home in silence.

I am more 'in tune' with God than religious during my middle years. We have a personal relationship, and I share with Him throughout the day. He's my constant companion, and I feel His presence even more closely in the days and weeks that follow. I find myself asking to be placed on prayer lists, and I make prayer lists of my own.

Barbara thoughtfully takes my email contacts and keeps friends apprised of my condition, allowing me a reprieve from having to engage in medical discussions. It's a compassionate gesture that most likely saves me from emotional collapse. A born storyteller, however, I eventually decide to take over reporting about my progress to friends and relatives personally.

I phone Derick Pindroh, a former student whom David refers

ACT II SCENE 1

to as "our boy." He says I'm too young to call him "son," Lord bless his sweet soul! Derick forever owns a portion of my heart, and we favor him with much affection. His strength and compassion help to sustain my spirit.

"Our boy," devastated by my update, responds on his blog with the following essay:

My Mentor and My Hero:

When I started high school, I didn't have anything going for me. In fact, I was three strikes down. I had just moved to Laurens, South Carolina, from Cleveland, Ohio, so I was a Yankee. Strike one. I was the new kid in town. Strike two. I was a preacher's kid. Strike three. I felt like I was doomed!

Then I discovered the wonderful world of theater! Our school was doing a production of "Up the Down Staircase," and I volunteered to do props and clean up the stage between acts. In doing so, I became enthralled with the costume closet! I was constantly trying on costumes and playing in a wheelchair used as a prop. The drama teacher, Miss Carnes, says she often wondered to herself: "Who is that strange little boy wearing all of the costumes and playing in the wheelchair?"

She didn't kick me out. Instead, she allowed me to become a part of the drama scene. She taught me to focus my creative 'muse,' if you will, and began to hone my dramatic skills. Over the next four years I blossomed into a fairly accomplished actor. Miss Carnes got married and became Mrs. Muse—fitting, don't you think? We developed a very close relationship—which continues today—and I consider her and her husband to be two of my closest friends.

Fast forward twenty years. I now live in Tennessee—Jimmi-Ann and David still live in South Carolina. I credit Jimmi-Ann with a lot of who I am today. She was my mentor and my 'muse.' And she was (and still is) a powerful encouragement to me.

About a month ago, she called to tell me that the doctor had found some cancerous cells and that she was going to be having surgery to remove them. Her spirit and her positive view on everything that was happening catapulted her from being just my mentor to being my hero! The surgery went well, and she is on the mend. Well, they discovered that the cancer has metastasized in the liver—but she is still extremely positive.

Here is a short segment from an email I got from her yesterday: *On July 8, I go for another CT scan. If the spot is smaller than the first scan, we will do nothing but keep an eye on it. If it is no longer there, praise God! I REALLY have been calm and peaceful about the whole thing . . . this experience will give me the chance to help other people. The future looks bright, and I have faith that all will be well.*

Do you see why she is my hero?

After a month of existing in a state of shock, the Warrior-Woman that surfaced during the initial diagnosis dons her armor and outfits herself to seize control of her destiny!

SCENE 2

My Script for Vibrant Living:
The Warrior's Arsenal ~ Twenty-One Weapons for Survival and Victory

*"Woman up! Gird your loins
and claim your power!"*
~ JIMMI-ANN

The actor in me surges forth like a tornado out of a phone booth!
I intentionally create the spotlight for my own healing!
As the leading character in the performance of my life, I am determined to live!

Warrior-Woman's Arsenal is crucial to survival and victory!

These armaments for wellness will evolve into a delightful way to approach living consciously:

The Power of Prayer

I carry God in my heart—always. I open up to fellow patients and "testify" in waiting rooms. Frequently, with my heart full, I wind up praying with them and for them. In return, they promise to include me in their prayers.

I have become aware that prayer is everywhere. While driving, I notice signs on church marques that include a number for prayer requests. There are dozens, and I call them all. I record the number in my journal each time I make a request. Six months later, I phone every one of them again, thankful that all those prayers have contributed to my personal miracle.

Hope and Belief

I never give up! As devastating as the prognosis is, I never give in to it—never own it. I consistently refer to it as *the* cancer and never claim it. Fear and Turbulence confront me, but I obstinately refuse to surrender.

Somehow, I resolutely fight Adversity and hold Faith close to me so that I will be able to triumph over Cancer. I believe that all will be well. The more I embrace Hope, the stronger Belief becomes. I stubbornly refuse to allow devious ambushes by terrible emotions to linger, and I stubbornly reject Defeat!

Doubt and Fear

Warrior-Woman is ambushed by reoccurring Doubt and Fear. My performance for others is stellar, yet I can't help but muse: *What if I can't get well? What if I die? What if I leave David?* The *What Ifs* flood my brain, though I want desperately to abandon being stalked by Anxiety. Intuition tells me I *can* beat Cancer if I can relinquish Foreboding, Anger, and Grief, who are also reoccurring antagonists.

My desire to eliminate the deepening shadows that haunt me becomes my prime directive.

It's sad that it's so very difficult to believe in Miracles and so easy to surrender Optimism to Fear. I take a determined breath; the tools for conquering Cancer are at my disposal, and the battle plans firm up.

Warrior-Woman is repeatedly ambushed by crippling emotions. However, I eventually perceive that *all the* characters in my saga are essential to the plot. One by one, Fear, Anger, Doubt, and Grief are conquered, and as they fall, the strength inherent in my body blossoms.

Every light reveals a shadow, and once a system is in balance it becomes a better-tuned, self-healing mechanism.

Once I embrace Trust and Acceptance and welcome *all challenges* coursing through me, they become insignificant players in my life because Love, the supreme and guiding light, emerges.

Uplifting Support of Family and Friends

I embrace the enfolding affection and strength of those close to me—the earthly angels whose compassion lightens my spirit and fuels my determination to survive. My family and friends help me realize that even as I confront Cancer, I can lift my wings and soar! Loving relationships are powerful remedies!

Medicine

I utilize just about every method available to combat the dreaded disease. Fear surfaces, screaming that Chemotherapy will wreak havoc upon my bodily systems. After much deliberation, I choose to employ the medicinal regimen; it becomes another weapon in my arsenal, an essential weapon to help me win the war. Every tool I use to fight Cancer will work harmoniously to facilitate my ultimate recovery.

Healing Foods

Medicine! Nutrition! Toxicity! Choice!

Organic whole foods act as medicine or nourishment for my body, while conventional foods can act as poison. How do you choose to employ food in your diet? Warrior-Woman swore fealty to the healing capabilities of nutrition.

I have presented evidence of the importance of natural foods and making healthy choices when seeking sustenance because they are a foundation for good health. Nutritional changes paired with vitamins, supplements, and digestive enzymes helped set the stage for my recovery. I choose recommended foods because they are integral to my arsenal for healthy living.

Stress Relief

I continue to seek unconventional approaches to wellness. Barbara joins me to take classes in meditation and sound therapy.

I look to energy healing, an ancient modality involving the act of moving and shifting energy in the body to support its natural capacity to . . . well . . . heal.

I resolve that pairing the power of organic foods with an energy-enhancing approach to wellness is a splendid idea.

Next, I conclude that a hypnotherapist might be helpful and schedule an appointment. I perform deep breathing exercises and listen to calming words as I settle into a state of profound relaxation during these sessions. My therapist helps further strengthen my visualization skills—a technique I use to help clear my body of *dis*-ease.

She helps me understand that Fear is sneaky and will return. I need to be aware, recognize its presence, and let it go. She suggests that every time Fear threatens me, I should visualize putting it inside a bubble and watch it float away to the edge of the universe where it will pop, evaporate, and disappear! What a pleasing image. It works very well and is a technique I continue to use to rid myself of unwanted thoughts.

After one of our sessions, an overwhelming sweetness leaves me limp, languid, feeling light as a feather, absolutely blissful, and I weep at sensations of enfolding, incomparable beauty.

I ask her what's happening, and the hypnotist tells me I'm deeply cherished. She says a vast amount of energetic love touched and supported me during the session. Programmed by society to question such things, it's initially difficult for me to believe until she continues.

She alleges that I have no idea how many lives I've positively affected during my lifetime and that these energetic resources have gathered now to help me when I need it most. She asserts that the life force of people whose lives I've influenced and persons whom I have yet to meet are loving, supporting, and helping me. She states that this combined energetic presence will stay with me and help me through the days to come as I fight Cancer.

I do know that I float for days, cocooned in the loving energy that lingers. Upon reflection, I believe the healing began with this God-incident.

Life Lesson #26: *Never doubt the effect you have made upon those whom you encounter.*

A long-lost friend, Amenie Schweizer, proves essential to my emotional and spiritual evolution. We'd worked together at *The Lost Colony* in 1980, and she comes back into my life just when I need her most—another bestowed God-Incidence.

A certified holistic health practitioner and life coach, Amenie is a cherished friend, and I'm forever grateful we've made a heart connection! Amenie uses alternative healing, life coaching, and visualization techniques to help me further alleviate Stress and release Fear.

She teaches me that fundamental elements of the human psyche include emotions, burdens, and ties to events and people from the past.

An intuitive, Amenie is a gifted healer and a facilitator for clearing and centering. I've been carrying old baggage that's been weighing me down, and she helps me release long-held emotions and wounds. My friend is instrumental in helping me relinquish the past so that I may live in the present. David and I are thankful to Amenie for the blessing she is in both of our lives.

The Power of Positivity

I welcome each day with positive intentions and choices. In the beginning, remaining in confident energy is difficult because I'm incessantly bombarded with Doubt, Fear, and *What Ifs*; they have become principal characters in my life's drama. However, the more I focus on Optimism, the easier my journey becomes.

The more I practice hopeful thinking, the less troubled I become. Positive intentions become elemental; I focus on being whole and well. I *know* I have to "get messages" to my subconscious, and I work at staying upbeat as a good way to begin to support this aspect of my battle! (I wouldn't be here today if I had dwelled on negativity and the doctor's diagnosis.)

The Advocacy of Words

The words a leading lady speaks reflect the essence of her character.

I recognize, more than ever, the power of language. Texts, books, song lyrics, and videos begin to inform my journey, and as I listen, journal, and read, my learning expands. It's as if messages of guidance arrive at just the right time in each of these varied forms. I realize that I should be very careful in choosing the words I think because negative self-description adversely affects my state of being.

I pay attention to these resources as they come into my awareness, and I begin to think, speak, and act from a place of greater awareness and understanding. This leads to the *Wall of Hope* I create by covering a section of our kitchen cabinets with timelines, affirmations, and prophecies, reminding me to remain positive and focused on my goals whenever I prepare an organic meal or waltz through the kitchen.

Say and Sing it Until You Believe It

Consistent repetition of what I want to be true is imperative to my healing. The more I repeat the outcomes I so desperately desire, the easier it is to believe. Repetition helps me manifest wellness by connecting me to my unconscious thoughts.

Music acts as a great healer. Repeating lyrics, melodies, and rhythms stimulates the brain, so singing about being healthy enhances my recovery. The vocalization of songs sends messages deep into my cells and into my subconscious. Recurring "well-being" song lyrics help pull me out of an emotional *flight or fight* mode and into relaxation, calmness, and belief.

Sometimes, as we wait for invasive tests after one of our "prayer sessions," I impulsively give voice to hymns, initiating impromptu sing-alongs!

My recovery is enhanced by acting and singing as if what I desire has already happened.

God-Incidences

God-Incidences are gateways to miracles; they're opportunities awaiting discovery! I become aware of miracles available for the taking and gratefully rejoice in accepting them.

Slowing Down

Forever rushing about in my chaotic world, I discover that "putting on the brakes" to slow down gives me time to become more aware of life itself. It turns out to be a most precious gift, allowing me the freedom and opportunity to recognize possibilities and miraculous pathways. Slowing down helps me stop living in the past and worrying about the future, resulting in a more comfortable life; I'm finally at ease in my own skin!

Living in the Present

Warrior-Woman finds the courage to let go of Distress and Worry.

No longer overly concerned about days gone by and days yet to come, I find myself much, much happier. It is as if my heart has been set free to truly *live* for the first time! Once I begin living in the present, life ultimately becomes wonderfully and joyfully harmonious.

Getting Out in Nature

Mother Earth is an excellent healer. Vitamin D is significantly boosted by sunshine. Getting outdoors, breathing fresh air, reflecting upon its beauty, and being grateful for all its glory projects peace and harmony. Going outside produces smiles and helps relieve Anxiety and Depression.

The Body in Motion

Warrior-Woman, bursting with newly discovered willpower, *imagines* herself flying off the sofa with enough energy to shake her bootie!

Walk! Get off your duff and walk!

I shuffle sluggishly down the country lane, huffing and puffing in the stiflingly oppressive South Carolina summer heat and humidity.

It's like an oasis in the desert when I see David's truck crest the hill and finally appear as he returns home from work. I'm sweltering, worn out, and dehydrated. Grinning and waving, I relax and anxiously await rescue!

Zooooooooom!

He doesn't stop!

He drives right past me!!

Abandoned! Rejected! Ditched!

Holy smokes! I'm about to swoon because of the heat and my long-neglected, unfit body, and he passes me by!

Warrior-Woman wilts further.

"Oh, look!" Thank heavens, the rascal's turning back!

His explanation extinguishes my agitation when he tells me I've lost so much weight that he—my own husband—didn't recognize me as he drove by!

Mercifully, when he glanced in the rearview mirror, he recognized my shaking finger!

Good gracious alive! Warrior-Woman is morphing into a Transformer!

My journey *is* going to prove to be the best thing ever!

As I'm hiking the next day, my son-in-law, James, passes me in his car while heading toward town. I chuckle—he's as clueless as David had been. I keep high-stepping toward fitness, laughing through tortured breathing as James backs up to pull alongside me to ask if I need a lift.

"Daddy, that was Jimmi-Mom . . . why didn't you stop?" my two young granddaughters in the back seat had asked him. I find it fascinating that these young children recognized my spirit while the two adults relied on my physicality.

As bad a shape as I'm in, the challenging endeavor of walking ignites an impressive lifestyle change in my fitness level. I suggest that if you are not exercising, the simple act of getting off the couch and moving can be the first step to a healthier life and outlook!

Exercise

Life-saving foods provide me with a significant energy boost. After my incision heals, I join the YMCA and begin a daily practice of swimming laps at six a.m. The early morning swims certainly challenge the warrior in this woman! Enhanced by walking, my stamina builds rapidly, and I become much stronger. Swimming had been an obsession during my youth, and rediscovering my passion for it is delightful—not only for its health benefits but for the memories it evokes.

Dance is another happy way I employ music and place exercise into my wellness program. I discover through my research that exercising and deep breathing can help destroy Cancer. Exercise helps get oxygen to the cellular level; cancer cells cannot live in an oxygenated environment.[6]

Humor, Chuckles, and Grins

"Laughs With Great Thunder" is a nickname gifted to me by a co-worker. It undeniably describes the resonance and force behind my laughter. I take great pleasure in giggling and encouraging others to engage!

Laughter increases our level of endorphins,[7] which are natural painkillers, and I resolve to chuckle more to deal with mental health and fatigue.

I know that author and peace advocate Norman Cousins used hilarity to recover from a painful, life-threatening disease. Cousins used good nutrition, vitamins, exercise, and laughter to create wellness. He believed that human emotions were basic to combatting illness and that merriment could help cure it. After realizing that ten minutes of deep belly chuckles left him pain-free for several hours, he'd isolate himself in a hotel room to watch funny movies and laugh. When discomfort returned, he'd switch on hilarious entertainment and laugh so the pain would retreat. He was convinced that he cured himself by laughing.

Laughing is one of my favorite things and I find it easy to incorporate as an element of my recovery.

Several years after winning the war on Cancer, I was introduced to Laughter Yoga, which combines laughter with yogic breathing techniques. Laughter Yoga International, a global movement for better health and happiness, fosters world peace through voluntary laughter.

I take a course to become an official instructor and use laughing exercises at the beginning of my classes to help students get oxygen to their brains to promote better focus. Some teachers allow students to use this method to release stress before tests and find they generally score higher grades.

I recommend deep belly laughter as a daily practice because it helps oxygenate the blood, reduce cortisol levels, improve focus, relieve stress, and makes you happy. In short, laughing is good for the soul.

Stepping Out—Breaking Out of Self-Imposed Isolation

Cabin fever strikes and sticks!

While well-wishers are welcome and embraced at our house, I realize I must get out and about.

Our home has a delightfully charming, therapeutic quality, but I decide that socializing will lessen my feelings of isolation and calm my persistent threat about that awful lurking character, Death.

Confinement or isolation is non-productive and depressing.

Stepping out becomes a happy distraction from the disease.

We celebrate at our favorite restaurant owned by a dear friend, Anita Baldwin. She lovingly directs me to bring her my organic foods, which she carefully prepares so we can enjoy being out socially. I'm delighted as I absorb the festive atmosphere and humbled by the affection that enfolds me as I drink warm water (because of the side effects of chemo) from an oversized margarita glass. Comforted by his favorite Mexican fare, David jokes and laughs with John, Anita's husband. My heart rejoices to see him so relaxed and having fun, a few minutes removed from our troubles. Being surrounded by the many earthly angels who care about us is a precious blessing.

Upon request, our local Waffle House takes my organic eggs and olive oil and scrambles them for me so we can occasionally enjoy a breakfast outing. Other eateries let me bring "a picnic" to dine out, and we appreciate the normality it brings back into our lives by allowing us an opportunity to get out and "play."

Distractive Action

Warrior-Woman discovers that focused activity is an essential element of healing.

Building, designing, and creating encourages attention directed outward rather than on oneself. Creative and enjoyable activities while pursuing wellness provide an excellent diversion.

The Artist Coop becomes a refuge as I take advantage of generating new canvases and watercolors to redecorate our home.

I'm also rediscovering myself through this artistic outlet, and it provides yet another place to "step out." School has been the center of my existence for so many years that I can't remember the last time I indulged in creating something for personal pleasure.

Focusing on a beloved activity while working toward my well-being helps get my mind off Trouble. Taking time to generate art proves meaningful because I lose myself in the process when creating, and all worrisome thoughts disappear.

Acceptance and Gratitude

Once I truly accept my troubles and become thankful for them, I give my Spirit what it requires to begin the healing process. Acceptance and Gratitude are elemental in allowing my body, mind, and soul the freedom to repair through the greatest healer, Love.

Love

Love is the most potent and essential tool in my arsenal. Compassion, Forgiveness, and Self-Acceptance are crucial to my healing. Through my soul journey, I discover that I must love myself completely. *Love. Myself. Completely.*

The step into loving myself unconditionally is the gateway. This access point allows me to stand strong in my conviction, grow through adversity, and maintain absolute faith that I will win my battle with Cancer.

Practicing self-love requires daily attention and intentional action. It demands that I release old thought patterns to step compassionately into my heart's gracious and abounding wisdom.

God-Incidences consistently appearing helps me form the foundation of my approach to recovery. Without the generous, loving relationships of friends and family and their constant care, David and I could not have borne the burden of the disease. Honing my skills and utilizing the tools that come into my life because of *the* cancer journey helps me build a place of safety and resiliency within myself.

Standing in the heart of the drama, my script perfectly memorized, I become the heroine of my journey, the star of the show, taking center stage, surrounded by God's light.

SCENE 3

Not Quite Ready to Believe:
Two More Miracles on the Road to Recovery

"I have to truly believe—with every cell in
my body—that I can beat this disease!"
~ JIMMI-ANN

The miracles—the never-ending miraculous God-Incidences—continue to reveal themselves, but I've been programmed to disbelieve and continue to pursue Courage and Trust.

I'm stuck, yet I desperately want to live!

Warrior-Woman will conquer General Chaos' invading minions, but I remain uncertain, believing I deserve to suffer before I can heal!

In my discussions with other terminal patients, I discover that this is a prevalent belief: *I am being punished for something . . . I was so terrible that the punishment must last a while.*

In retrospect, I sense that if this thought had never surfaced, I would have healed even more quickly. Trusting in possibilities instead of inevitability is basic to recovery.

Life Lesson #27: *God is love; He does not want us to suffer.*

I'm convinced that thoughts prolong sickness.

Constantly working diligently to remain positive, I question how I might control my unconscious thoughts.

Scientists are just beginning to learn how powerful the brain is, how every cell in our body has memory, and how each cell is affected by our thoughts and beliefs. Therefore, it's crucial for me to redirect feelings that are preventing my recovery.

This delves into quantum physics, but I'll discuss that later.

It's no coincidence that a friend knows a lay preacher willing to anoint me with oil and lay on hands as he prays for me. This ritual for the sick is a practice of atonement and a conduit for God's devotion. It's an outward, visible sign of an inward, spiritual blessing. Anointment and the laying on of hands are considered God's gifts.

I want both.

I'm given the minister's phone number, and I call him. We chat briefly, and he says he's willing to pray with me but reveals that I'm already healed.

Stubborn, I haven't yet reached a place where I can truly believe. Lacking faith, I don't want to take any chances! The more prepared I am for the role, the more confidence I will demonstrate!

He agrees to meet with me where he's working.

Three miracle-seeking women prepared for an extraordinary prayer meeting join two carpenters who are reverends working on a construction site. They're completing a new housing development several towns away, and we commence the ultimate private prayer meeting in an unfinished living room!

We pray, sing hymns, and cry.

I lift my arms in praise and express a multitude of emotions as oil and hands are laid on to revive my health.

Intoxicated with the vibrant power of pure affection, this experience is life-changing in that I feel His presence completely.

Exulted and exhausted, we prepare to leave, but I'm stopped as I start out the door.

"*You* are a healer," my new friend says, astonishing me. "You now have the responsibility to go out and heal others," he continues, placing a vial of oil in my hands. He explains how to replenish the oil once I use it and sends me on my way.

We drive home, dazed but overwhelmed with tenderness.

Words cannot express how glorious and thankful I feel.

After relating the day's events to David, I confess how surprised I was to be given the oil and told I'm a healer.

He grins mischievously.

"What?" I ask him.

"Of course, you're a healer! I've always known that!" David raises his eyes to heaven, gesturing to me that I need to believe in myself as much as he believes in me.

"What are you talking about?" I ask incredulously.

"Look at what you do with children."

(Dramatic pause!)

Well, knock me over with a feather!

I never think of my teaching as healing, but upon reflection, I realize it has that effect.

Isn't it strange that we need prompts to see how others perceive us in order to see ourselves more clearly?

I'm learning, through this evolution, that I'm more than I ever believed myself to be.

Life Lesson #28: You are unique in all the world; open your eyes and recognize your gifts; accept and use them gratefully.

An interesting aside about the oil: The reverend told me to replenish it with organic olive oil, to ask God to bless it, and to use it to heal. I can't help but smile at the thought that the oil is organic!

I arise early, welcoming a glorious new day, make my teas, and head for the porch to enjoy the splendor of the morning.

When I open the door, Buzz, our cat, looking like the king of the jungle, presents me with a trophy.

It's a dead bird at his feet.

I can tell he's very proud of his prowess.

Though my first instinct is to scold him, I refrain. He's a cat, and cats do what cats do.

Endeavoring to be nonjudgmental, I choose not to judge Buzz. Instead, I praise him for being a mighty cat, let him into the house, close the door, and pick up the dead wren.

I hold it, feeling helpless—what a horrible way to start my day.

I decide to bury the tiny bird and start down the steps.

Suddenly, I freeze.

I remember what the reverend said about my ability to heal.

Can I?

We live in the middle of twenty-eight acres, but I look around in case someone is watching.

I take a deep breath and begin to call for divine help on behalf of this little bird.

I plead that the feathered creature might be saved as I cry and keep my hands on its poor little body.

Eventually, I begin to sing the old hymn, *"His Eye Is on The Sparrow and I Know He Watches Me."*

I keep at it for a good little while.

Nothing.

Feeling foolish, I give up, place the bird on the railing, and sit down, heartbroken and weary.

I feel terrible.

I feel awful.

I gasp.

I do a double-take.

I hold my breath.

Is that movement I see?

With a bent, wet neck, this little bird struggles to its feet and peers about!

Now I have goosebumps!

It manages a few steps, shakes itself, and looks around.

After a little while, it flies to a nearby tree and begins to chirp.

Astonished, I stand in my two-sizes-too-big nightshirt, listening to birdsong and weeping. I raise my arms to the sky and drink in the beauty and glory of nature, in awe of Divine power.

I have been gifted another miracle!

I've been given another clear sign that anything is possible!

I didn't heal that bird—God did.

That bird might have been stunned the whole time, although I didn't feel a heartbeat. Nevertheless, I know I witnessed a Miracle, and that Spirit was teaching me as it worked through me . . .

Life Lesson #29: *God is all-powerful; it is* our *soul responsibility to have faith.*

I ponder the proverb *Physician, heal thyself* found in Luke 4:23. Although the moral of the adage is the advice to focus on our own shortcomings rather than criticizing faults in others, it has a new additional meaning to me. I believe God is the infinite energy in all things; He is everywhere and a part of everything. There is an element of God in the birds, the trees, the ocean, and every grain of sand. Therefore, He is part of me. That inner voice, that God-part, can do anything because it is *of* God. To me, *Physician, heal thyself* also means that through the grace of the One who lives internally, I can assist in my own healing.

Life Lesson #30: *There are powerful dormant abilities within each of us waiting to be discovered; believing in and accessing these gifts is a birthright.*

SCENE 4

Quantum Physics Annihilates the Inner Monologue:
The Gift of Self-Acceptance and Self-Love

"Remember, you're unique in all the world . . .
just like everyone else!"
~DAVID

*I*f you know me, when I mentioned that I'd discuss quantum physics, your eyebrows surely would have risen, and you would have grinned!

I am an artist, not a mathematician. I am neither scientist nor theologian, but I feel obligated to discuss the importance of quantum physics to my recovery.

Soon after our tofu adventure, Barbara asks if I've seen the motion picture *What the Bleep Do We Know!?*[8]

I think she's trying to be funny by making up the name, but she explains she saw the film several years ago and believes it might hold some answers for me. She gives me a copy of the movie, gifting me with yet another God-Incidence.

David and I begin to watch the video, knowing only that it's a documentary woven with a storyline about the metaphysical world of quantum physics. It looks at science, spirituality, and their possible link. I'm puzzled by some of the concepts as I watch. During technical sections, I stop the movie several times to ask for explanations and see whether I'm understanding it correctly. David clarified the confusing segments.

The movie suggests that every single cell in our body has intelligence, and each one has memory.

All the cells work the way we direct them to—with our words, actions, and thoughts. We tell our cells how to perform through our behavior. Oprah and Dr. Phil instruct us to stop the constant negative internal monologue that many of us play; the connection to cell memory is undoubtedly their rationale.

I suffered from chronic pain for nine years prior to a hip replacement in 2003. The negative narration inside my head became even more vicious due to my constant physical discomfort. Chronic pain is grueling—spiritually, mentally, and physically. I couldn't participate in activities I enjoyed. I became sedentary, gained weight, and didn't like the person I'd become. Therefore, I secretly and continuously demeaned myself.

The negative self-talk became brutal, and I still engage in it years after having received the new hip and long after the pain subsided.

The movie proposes that our cells work as we instruct them with our words, actions, and thoughts.

It makes me contemplate ideas on a level I've never considered: What if our cells actually understand our thoughts?

What if we control our cells with our conscious *and* unconscious observations?

Since I felt so unworthy for such a long time, does that mean I conjured up cancer unknowingly?

I suddenly make a startling connection, which most certainly feels true: *Because I felt crappy about myself, I developed colon cancer!*

As David and I continue watching the video, my senses are most jarred by the scene focused on Japanese water experiments. The

ACT II SCENE 4

tests, conducted by Masaru Emoto, a Japanese researcher whose published book *The Hidden Messages in Water,* illustrate the findings of his worldwide study.[9] His work convinces me that my thoughts affect everything in and around me, and his experiments profoundly change my life.

Water, the source of all life as we know it, is fundamentally important to every life form. Human energy is vibrational – all matter is vibrational. Mr. Emoto set out to prove that thoughts, words, and music affect the structure of molecules.

That brings us to his experiments: Mr. Emoto conducted his research and produced evidence that words influence water. He filled several vessels with water drawn from a natural spring and set one aside as a control sample. A Buddhist monk blessed one jug, and Emoto wrote different words or phrases on the other containers and left them overnight.

The next day, he took samples from each one, froze them, and looked at single molecules under a microscope.

The control sample looked exactly like a six-sided frozen water molecule should look. Unexpectedly, the water that the monk blessed was six-sided but looked like a beautiful, lacy, iridescent snowflake. Positive phrases he'd written on the jugs, such as *I adore you, You are wonderful,* and *You are magnificent,* produced six-sided ice crystals. Though varied, the intentions written on each resulted in a different yet exquisite snowflake pattern!

Water has very flexible properties; its physical form conforms to its environs or vessels. According to Mr. Emoto, not only does the physical appearance of water change to adapt to its environment, but its molecular shape changes with differences in energy vibrations, too!

To prove his theory that water literally reflects its environment, Mr. Emoto wrote the equivalent of *I hate you; I am going to kill you,* on the last jug.

The result is mindboggling!

The frozen molecule was not six-sided.

It was not iridescent.

It was not beautiful.

The water molecule with the negative intention was ugly and misshapen, and the color of antifreeze that leaks from a car.

His work suggests that our words and thoughts most definitely affect our bodies because we're composed of vibrating particles.

This notion stops me cold and shakes me to the core.

Having bombarded myself with negative energy for such a very long time, I immediately made the connection that disapproving thoughts adversely influence my health. After all, if the adult human body is composed of over fifty percent water, and I criticized myself for years and years and years, is there any wonder that *dis*-ease developed?

This concept shakes me to the core and changes my perception of *dis*-ease. I recognize its wisdom and embrace it.

The morning after watching *What the Bleep*, while preparing twig tea, I accidentally spill loose tea twigs all over the countertop. Falling into my old pattern of self-criticism, I think: *You stu*—but catch myself and change my thought to *you stu–pendously wonderful woman! Everybody makes mistakes!* I refuse to call myself stupid anymore, and thus begins the revolutionary idea of loving Jimmi-Ann!

I clean the mess on the counter and clean up my internal monologue.

From that day forward, after learning about those experiments, I consciously decided that I prefer my water molecules to be iridescent and beautiful, so I practice being as kind and loving to myself as I have been to others.

I no longer criticize myself as I did when I gave my love away to those dear to me and even those I chanced to encounter. Now, as

ACT II SCENE 4

I embrace positive self-esteem, I work to think thoughts that will keep my molecules happy.

I was so unkind to myself. I criticized myself. Self-affection had been abandoned and forgotten. I secretly demonstrated the exact opposite of the concepts I teach students about self-worth.

Stunned to learn that loving myself is the greatest gift of all, I realize that by embracing *unconditional self-love*, the volume I generate to share with others is boundless.

Through the sickness, I realize I've been criticizing God. I am His creation; how dare I express contempt for myself?

Self-compassion makes my existence so much easier. Believing in my worthiness proves eye-opening and liberating; it brings lasting peace, easiness, and deep joy to all aspects of life.

It's heartbreaking that I waited to let tragic circumstances and a death sentence scare me into seeing myself as a wonderfully incredible human *Being*.

My advice to others: *Adore yourself!*

Never doubt your worth or the effect you have upon those you encounter.

Have affection for who you are!

Remind yourself of your self-ardor often!

Placing yourself *first* is not ego.

Placing yourself *first* is *not* selfish.

Placing yourself first allows you to flourish, live life to its fullest, empathize with others, and be much more available for them.

Life Lesson #31: *God's gifts of self-love and self-acceptance become easier with daily practice.*

Recently, I've concluded that my hip replacement was a God-Incident because it helped me release a decade of chronic pain three years before *the* cancer diagnosis, which in turn allowed me to embark on my wellness journey. Otherwise, I would have been so depleted and weak that recovery from the disease could not have happened. Again, what we perceive as adversity is often, in hindsight, a blessing.

Once more, the most challenging concept for me was making the paradigm shift away from self-criticism to self-love. Always a sensitive, compassionate caregiver, I prioritized everyone else as more significant, placed more value on others, and put everyone else first and myself consistently last.

I believe that women, especially, tend to follow this pattern because it's been bred into us for generations. We've allowed responsibilities, guilt, and pain to distract us from loving ourselves. Many people, caught up in emulating others and seeking what others have, end up feeling worthless, inadequate, and miserable. Why not rejoice instead in the miracle of our existence and do our best to emulate our loving Deity?

Life Lesson #32: *Strive to become a living example of God's love.*

I learned that when I value and accept myself in loving terms, I'm rewarded with boundless light and kindness to share with the world. So, loving myself becomes fundamental to my healing.

Think about it—every single individual is born extraordinary.

Brilliant. *Really* think about it!

Every single one of us has been extraordinary our entire lives! Although I teach this to my students, I never believed it about myself! Now, I know it's essential that this is something each of us understand and accept.

Life Lesson #33: *The greatest gift of all is unconditional self-love and self-acceptance.*

Life Lesson #34: *Through love, miracles manifest.*

SCENE 5

Building Blocks for My *Wall of Hope*: Timelines, Affirmations, and Prophesies

" . . . and these are words to live by!"
~ JIMMI-ANN

I create a timeline and post it on my kitchen cabinet door. Encouraged upon seeing it as I prepare our organic meals, I gradually begin adding more words to elevate my spirit. I nickname several cupboards my *Wall of Hope*; they remain a part of our home and a reminder of my incredible journey and my need to stay rooted in the present as I look toward the future.

Timeline:
August 2005
Focus on being cancer-free!
Chemotherapy is my friend.
Chemotherapy is my friend.
No adverse effects from the chemo!

October 2005: No cancer on CT scan—Stop chemo

December 18, 2005, Wedding Anniversary: Christmas is glorious! *I am cancer-free!*

> July 2006: Celebrate July Fourth on Outer Banks—better than ever!
>
> July 2007: Entire family on the beach!
>
> December 18, 2013: Thirtieth wedding anniversary!
>
> December 18, 2023: Fortieth wedding anniversary!
>
> December 18, 2033: Fiftieth wedding anniversary!

I placed this timeline on the cabinet door after booking our trip for the next Fourth of July. Rarely one to make lists or even write down goals; I'm blazing new territory. I compose affirmations and positive declarations of *hoped-for-truths* and add them to the cabinets, along with cards and good wishes from friends. I peruse my wall several times a day for inspiration. Many deadlines are met; I'm told chemo might be working in October! The family beach celebration occurs *a whole year ahead of schedule!*

Barbara gifted me with the book *Miracles* by Stuart Wilde, which became the most significant piece of writing I encountered during this period.[10] Wilde's wise words help me understand that I'm learning a new way to think and that this is precisely what I need to help me stand firm in my new convictions. Inspired by the book, I adopt his *"Understanding the Nature of Beliefs"* as my wellness plan to help illustrate how I'll tackle the obstacles set before me. Such a plan gives me hope, guidance, purpose, and strength, filling me with gratitude for Mr. Wilde.

Wellness Plan

I am cancer-free.

God-Spirit lives inside me, so God is a part of me.

I am infinite because my soul is infinite.

God-Spirit is Love.

Love gives me whatever I believe; I believe I am cancer-free.

I am a part of the living spirit named Love; I was placed on this planet to live, learn, and love.
I am not my intellect, feelings, or body; I am without boundaries because of divine Love.

Love is with me for eternity.

What I manifest for myself is mine because I conceive it through Love.

I am worthy and deserving!

I am worthy and deserving!

When we believe, God gifts us with miracles because miracles are part of our loving spirit.

God-Spirit lives in everyone. God-Spirit lives through me.

I am cancer-free.

The timeline and wellness plan look lonely on the cupboard, so I expand it by filling the space with affirmations, prayers, and cards:
I am beautiful. I am strong. I am infinite. I can make miracles happen!
After years of derogatory internal dialogue, what a fantastic new way to perceive myself!

Logic prevents miracles!
Believe!
If I had applied the *logic* of the experts, I would not be here today!

My mantra:
I am clear, I am clean, I am cancer-free!

ACT II SCENE 5

Here's another affirmation that states what I now believe as truth:
All things are possible through the Love of God! I am Jimmi-Ann. I am valuable, I am worthy, I am Love. I am open and receptive to my best and highest good.

Additional statements that become part of my *Wall of Hope*:
I try to remember to ask this about all the choices I make:
If this is not for my best and highest good, show me what is.

**All that we are is the result of what we have thought.
The mind is everything. What we think, we become.
~ The Buddha**

I use a five-by-six-inch canvas to create a painting with these words—another reminder to think *right* thoughts. What we think, we become. This goes back to the idea of quantum physics: *All creation begins with thought—the power of mind-action is thought.*

**Spread love wherever you go.
Let no one ever come to you without leaving happier.
~ Mother Teresa**

These words I journal become my truth:
*Regard everyone with compassionate eyes.
Bless everyone with the Love that you are.
Do your best to take Jesus's place until He returns.
Miracles happen when we complete our past—then we understand that love is everywhere, and the whole world becomes sparkling new. We attract what we are being.
The first thing is to be happy.
Be happy no matter what . . . then all else falls into place.
Be happy.*

This prayer of thanksgiving provides a way to begin believing and understanding the power of Love: *"Thank You for helping me understand that Love blesses me, and Love blesses through me. I am healthy and whole in body, mind, and soul because You created me to enjoy learning and living as a Being on this planet. I am so very grateful for my life and Your love. Thank you for the blessing of Love moving through me and out to others. Amen."*

To believe something without a doubt, I had to create the attitude that it has *already* happened and to make what I long for a part of my life *before* it manifests.

Act as if what I want has already happened!

This is *very* important—to act as if desires have already been achieved!

Love is. God is Love. Our role is to love. God is Love. Love is.

Through His power, I am empowered to assist in my own healing.

I journaled These essential words; they became my truth: *Regard everyone with compassionate eyes. Bless everyone with the Love that you are.*

We heal from the inside out!

My ability to use food, exercise, and positive energy to recover certainly brings this point home!

A quote from my journal describes my support system: *"Without my angels, I would not have survived."*

Blessings to my friends and loved ones, my angels, who help me remember that I have wings! *"Family and friends are earthly angels who elevate me and remind me to unfurl my wings when burdened."*

Helen Keller, a hero and shining example of God's miracles coming out of darkness, said: *"Keep your face to the sunshine, and you cannot see the shadow."*

This is a difficult concept to learn, but here's a journal entry I made in September 2005: "Once I learned to *love* myself and let go of my *fears* and *disapproving* inner monologue, I became powerful

ACT II SCENE 5

beyond imagination. *Fear and negativity cripple us, limit us, and keep us from becoming who we were born to be."*

I invented a 'device' inspired by the Japanese water experiment. Here's an enlarged copy of the postage-stamp-sized *Cancer Patch* that I wore over my heart for a week before the surgery-determining PET scan.

You will learn of it in ACT III Scene 4:

A Strong, Powerful, New Me . . .
Angered by a Third Surgeon, I Invent the Cancer Patch!

> **No need for surgery. The tumors are gone.**

Hallelujah, it works!

The PET scan undoubtedly surprises the
surgeon because the tumors *are* gone!

The words that cover my Wall of Hope help me stay in positive energy and encourage my transformative journey every step of the way!

SCENE 6
It's All About Perspective:
Chemotherapy is Not a Wake or a Funeral!

"Oh boy! Chemotherapy gives me a splendid reason to wear a costume!"
~ JIMMI-ANN

*E*leven weeks after colon surgery and seven and a half weeks into *FoodWisdomRx*, I am to begin chemotherapy treatments.

My family doctor orders blood tests to set a baseline for comparison after chemo. She is as eager as I am to get pre-chemo results to see if my organic eating and exercise endeavors have been effective; she gives me hope. Optimistic about my chances for survival, she draws more than twenty vials of blood and tests me for things beyond my ken.

Love, determination, right-eating, movement, and all the rest are moving this fighting Warrior toward conquering the dreaded antagonist!

On the morning of my first chemical cocktail, this hopeful doctor conveys fantastic news: My extensive bloodwork has come back normal on every test! My immune system is in perfect working order even though it has been out of whack for the past ten years! After "cleaning up my act" for fifty-seven days, my body's primed for what is to come because it's now functioning as intended!

My doctor's incredible communication validates that everything I've been doing is right! Sixty-seven pounds lighter since the virus at Christmas—forty-two of those pounds lost since I began eating to live and moving my body—I feel better than I have in years! Even though the blood tests assessing my systems are perfect, and I've cut out sugar, dairy, meat, and caffeine—*the* cancer remains.

Although I'm fearful of exposing my body to chemical bombardment, I make sure that I'm fighting with every tool available by consenting to chemotherapy.

It's challenging to act as if I'm already healed, but I'm making progress toward believing it's possible.

Life Lesson #35: *Proper food is medicine.*

Why am I surprised by my test results?

I'd read in a medical journal about a study on children who consumed conventional foods and how testing revealed numerous toxins in their blood. Researchers then placed them on an organic diet for three days and retested them. Results showed their blood to be pure and clean. Three days on organic foods and the miracle that is the human body cleans out the contaminants in every single child!

As a teacher, I've witnessed first-grade girls start their periods and little boys develop breasts. I now realize that these students consumed over-processed, non-organic foods containing growth hormones and other contaminants. It is exceedingly sad for me to finally comprehend just how over-processed and potentially dangerous our foods have become.

"The doctor of the future will give no medicine but will interest his patient in the care of the human frame, diet, and in the cause and prevention of disease," Thomas Edison stated long ago, as he was troubled about healthcare options throughout his lifetime. I know now that he was right; eating natural foods can have the same positive effects as medicine.

Life Lesson #36: *The human body is a miraculous instrument with the ability to cleanse and heal itself if treated as a holy vessel.*

Warrior-Woman gleefully approaches the first chemo treatment after receiving her extraordinary lab report but insists that Barbara and David let her handle the chemotherapy sessions alone. I promise to ask for help if I need their company, knowing they both need time for self-care and that sitting around waiting for me would have been loving but unproductive. Besides, the first infusion lasts four-and-one-half hours, and consecutive ones even longer. They reluctantly accede to my wishes.

The chemo considered best for me comes in six-packs, and I firmly determine that a second six-pack will *not* be necessary; I adamantly refuse to believe I'll be on chemo for the rest of my life!

I refuse to act as if I'm attending my own wake, and I step into the scene of chemo sessions as a performer. Costumed in a Hulk camp shirt, a feather boa, and a large, flowered picture hat, I resolve to brighten the scene. After all, I'm not attending a funeral!

I bring daisies to give to the other patients to urge a smile. I carry art supplies, a novel, magazines, and legal snacks from the food program. My Hulk shirt is a tongue-in-cheek tribute to Stan Lee's Bruce Banner—I won't be bombarded with radiation, but the chemicals are going to change me, and I decide to imagine myself as strong as the Marvel Comics character.

Second thoughts about my crazy attire cause me to hesitate before opening the door to the oncologist's waiting room, but I forge ahead.

To my surprise, no one even grins—my dramatic entrance is wasted!

I take my medicine, work on art, and don't give my clothes a second thought until three weeks later when I return for my second infusion. Again, I dress in the Hulk shirt and am laden with posies and supplies to create artsy gifts for my fellow patients. This time, I leave my newly crafted feathered hat in the car, having decided it wasn't valued during my first visit.

"Where's the hat?" the receptionist queries in a monotone. Her eyes meet mine as she raises one eyebrow.

Bravo!

Hooray! Theatrical Appreciation!

I retrieve my chapeau and dress accordingly for each remaining appointment.

Spiraling out of control for years, I'm finally in command!

It's a strange way to feel with Cancer as a constant companion, but my belief that I'll be cured continues to intensify.

Life Lesson #37: *Miracles are available for the asking and the believing; believing is the challenging part.*

A former student's father is the physician who surgically inserts a port over my heart that delivers the medicinal infusions.

A therapeutic port accommodates the foundation of a small tube inserted into a blood vessel to carry chemicals directly into the heart, offering a simple and almost painless way to dispense chemotherapy drugs. Without this process, each chemotherapy session would require needle punctures to draw blood for tests and an attached I-V for infusion of the medicine. I detest the thought of an I-V because, with it, every treatment would have to be injected into different veins in either my hands or arms.

Administering the drugs becomes a much easier process because of this method, both because it delivers the inserted drugs directly and because injections can cause the collapse of blood vessels over time. The port allows each chemotherapy treatment to begin with a fairly painless stick into the apparatus, and that's it.[11]

The device makes a small lump above my right breast that itches almost constantly. I had it removed after my recovery, and though it leaves a small scar, I consider it a war injury and a beauty mark, reminding me that every method I chose to fight *the* cancer ultimately led to success.

The meds administered are *Eloxatin* (*Oxaliplatin* injection) and *Avastin*. The two drugs, new at the time, attack *only* the cancer lesions. The following day, I'm to take *Xeloda* in the a.m. and *Compazni* in the p.m., both chemotherapy pills that together attack *every* cell in the body as per traditional chemo. The two tablets are to be taken daily for two weeks, and mercifully, I will be off everything for one week. Then, I repeat the entire process.

From my journal, early August 2005: The First Chemotherapy Infusion . . . During the first four-and-one-half hour infusion, I'm aware of a tingling in my feet and fingers. It goes away, but later, I become very warm several times. The nurse tells me it's just the medicine, not a hot flash.

I gulp some water, then my throat closes up and feels gravelly . . . I need to take it slowly when drinking.

I wash my hands with tap water, and it's uncomfortably cold. I have to avoid cold things for about two weeks following the drip.

Next, I think I'm getting a headache, but it never materializes. Instead, it just floats in and out around my temples and behind my eyes.

My chemotherapy nurse says it's likely that the palms of my hands and soles of my feet will turn red, dry out, and crack. She suggests Bag Balm for soothing relief.

At home later . . . I feel disconnected and emotional. I need to stop and ground myself. I started to tear up three times this evening, and there's a terrific, burning pain behind my eyes. The tears cause dreadful throbbing . . . I retrieve peppermint oil to place on my temples for headache relief.

ACT II SCENE 6

I will endeavor not to cry until this effect wears off, reportedly in about a week, even though it will be difficult since I've always cried at the drop of a hat—for happiness and any number of reasons.

I cook supper, and a cold radish 'burns' my fingers as I prepare a salad. This cold intolerance should dissipate within fifteen days. I have no problem eating, and I do so, but slowly, after my gulping of water episode. The twig tea doesn't quite reach room temperature, and the cold edge reminds me to warm my drinks.

Later, I grab a couple of almonds as David eats salted mixed nuts. After two chews, I'm horrified as it feels as if my jaws are locking. I begin to cry, and the pain behind my eyes becomes excruciating. Is this a reaction to salt?

Shattered, I decide to go to bed thinking I'll sleep really well.

David heads to the pharmacy for the chemo pills since I didn't feel like stopping for them after the infusion.

I hope I can maintain my positive attitude.

My sudden fear of withering into a brown leaf and being blown away does not happen. I'm following my energetic healer's advice to place negative thoughts inside a bubble and watch them float out to the edge of the universe, where I watch them burst and disappear.

The Pills: At home . . . The pills are not horrible. They don't cause nausea, constipation, or diarrhea, but I just don't feel like myself.

Sometimes, it's as if I'm without sensation, just a numb observer, watching what is happening to me.

The worst reaction remains the after-effects of the medicinal drip because when I become emotional and tear up, it now causes a severe headache along with the burning at the back of my eyes. I try to stop letting my feelings get the best of me, and I stop crying abruptly due to the piercing discomfort.

The burning eyes associated with my emotions vanish after a week. I am convinced that the adverse effects are due to the drip rather than

STAGE 4 TO CENTER STAGE!

the pills—anything cold affects my fingers and throat—even tap water induces pain. However, I discovered that when I use hot water, there's no constricting of my veins. Mercifully, the discomfort from temperature disappears two weeks following the infusion.

As forewarned, thin skin on my feet and hands develops and is another distressing effect of my reactions to the chemo.

On the Tuesday following the first drip, I experience uncomfortable stiffness in my muscles. I assume it might be due to hiking and the Tai Chi classes I took on Friday, Saturday, and Sunday following the first chemo treatment on Thursday.

We may never know . . .

SCENE 7

Road Trip the Day After My First Chemotherapy Treatment: *A Most Significant Pathway to Recovery is Revealed*

> "Go on Roxanne's retreat and try to 'forget' the cancer for a few days. Go with Barbara and have another grand adventure!"
> ~ DAVID

*I*nconceivable! Unbelievable! Incredible!

I embark on a retreat to Roanoke, Virginia, the morning after the first chemo treatment that helps me relax, focus on my inner voice, face Fear, and welcome Acceptance.

Barbara drives us to Asheville, and we crowd into Roxanne's van for the trip. The vehicle is filled with food for about forty people, cooking utensils, and five women's personal belongings for a long weekend. Astounded that we can cram the whole lot inside the vehicle and still manage to breathe, we travel with our coach, Roxanne's twin sister, Rosie, and another of Roxanne's clients.

Energized with high expectations, we hit the road for pleasure and instruction.

We giggle and laugh through the majestic mountains, and traveling together becomes a bonding, illuminating experience as Roxanne keeps up an informative and entertaining running commentary. I lament later that I should have taken notes, but at the same time rejoice in newfound friendships!

I feel a little off, but not enough to slow me down too much. With companions who watch over me, making sure I'm adjusting suitably to the trip and the after-effects of the medicine, I manage the weekend very well. Occasionally, I feel numb—as if I'm observing my life rather than participating in it. However, I never suffer any of the dire consequences I imagined during the diagnosis back in June.

The weekend proves to be a wonderful, life-changing experience.

I almost chickened out at the last minute! Well, for heaven's sake, I took my first chemo treatment yesterday!

I could have stayed home and felt sorry for myself all weekend. I'm so glad I resolved that self-pity was counterproductive. David would have supported me had I remained at home. When he wisely counseled me to go have fun in the mountains, he recognized that the trip would provide normalcy during the weekend. And this *normalcy* proves to be another pivotal point in my recovery.

Somehow, I found the fortitude to never once bemoan, "Why *me?*"

I simply went to work and changed my state of affairs.

Roxanne and Rosie prepare all the meals for the retreat, and their cooking is incredible! Barbara and I are initiated as impromptu kitchen staff for three days, and the experience serves as cooking lessons. We wash, chop, slice, dice—even learn to matchstick. Delighted to acquire fascinating information about foods, their preparation, and Roxanne's program, we're even more ecstatic at the prospect of sampling their meals. I continue to be very careful with temperature and avoid excessive "burning" of my fingers or mouth.

I'd never eaten kale (until beginning the food plan), but I learned that it's a superstar among vegetables. An excellent source of vitamins A, K, B6, and C, calcium, potassium, copper, and manganese, kale

ACT II SCENE 7

is low in calories and carbohydrates and perfect for weight loss. It can even possibly lower the risk of several types of cancer.

Roxanne infuses a bit of garlic in toasted sesame oil, adds the kale, and turns the leafy veggie over until it's a bright green. A simple but delicious recipe, she teaches us how to stack kale leaves, roll them like a cigar, and then cut very, very thin slices for preparation. Toss on a few toasted pumpkin seeds for garnish, and you have a fantastic addition to any meal.

Eventually, I added a little onion and shredded cabbage to Roxanne's recipe to include two more vegetables in this delectable dish. It's so tasty I can't get enough of it, and it has become one of David's favorites—he—who never liked greens unless they were in a salad. And salads, oh my, oh my . . . Roxanne shares several wonderful salad recipes that can be refrigerated for up to five days.

While consuming these scrumptious salads at mealtimes, Barbara and I giggle that we'll probably have difficulty not gobbling them up as soon as they're concocted.

However, we're reminded that slow, thoughtful eating with proper mastication lets us realize we're full before we overindulge. Many schoolteachers, you see, tend to *inhale* their food at lunchtime to have time to take care of personal business before the next class begins. Guilty of that terrible practice at *every* meal, I find that inhaling food is a hard habit to break!

Eating very slowly and chewing properly delivers digestive enzymes from the mouth to the food, and prolonged chewing assists in the absorption of nutrients. We learn to eat slowly and chew thoroughly, filling us up more quickly, resulting in better digestion and less intake.

Surprisingly, because of my former aversion, I become very, very, very best friends with a particular soybean product when the sisters use it to create a vegan chocolate mousse. The recipe's main ingredient is tofu, and we watch with eager anticipation as the silky dish is concocted—we can't suppress our excitement at being able to devour chocolate!

Roxanne spoons a small amount for each of us to taste, and oh my, oh my, oh my—the dessert is delightfully delectable!! It's amazingly creamy and oh *sooooooo* chocolaty—Rosie, Barbara, and I could have eaten the entire batch made for everyone. But Roxanne makes us wait until mealtime for a more satisfying serving.

Rosie manages to highjack the spoon while we student "cooks" pathetically use our fingers to swipe the remaining bits of chocolate cream clinging to the bowl! This is one recipe we'll definitely reproduce at home!

Barbara and I room together, confide in each other, and have a wonderful time just *Being*.

The mountains are exquisite and take on a holy ambiance.

We crave peace. We crave beauty. We crave distance from the turmoil our lives have become, and the spectacular Blue Ridge Mountains set that scene. Deep in the heart of the mountains, our spirits open to the comforting calm. We're content, and it's a blessing to take it easy and perhaps forget about my situation for a little while.

Life Lesson #38: *The planet is glorious! Offer appreciation and gratitude for all of creation!*

Again, taking a "normal" break during chaos becomes the best thing that could have possibly happened. Thanks to my beloved for being so wise; though seeing me leave right after the infusion was difficult, David knew it was for the best.

A few days earlier, when Roxanne called and asked if we'd like to attend this retreat, I had a feeling that the interlude would become another beautiful God-Incident, and I turn out to be right.

ACT II SCENE 7

Lesson #39: *Getting out in nature is comforting, calming, uplifting, and healing; make embracing nature a priority.*

Barbara and I attend several classes together:

Tai Chi class in the mornings and evenings at the edge of the forest is soothing and relaxing. The slow movement and calming focus help me reduce the myriad thoughts ever crashing through my mind.

We attend guided meditations surrounded by the magnificence of nature, and I discover peace deep within my heart.

We hike trails and bask in the splendor of the natural environment.

We enjoy instruction in sound therapy.

I take things easy, declining a few classes to rest instead.

I take pleasure in my companion's excitement about her additional activities.

I journal and sketch.

We delight in consuming the sisters' excellent repasts.

As Barbara and I continue to observe how these two professional cooks delight in their craft, we learn additional methods and techniques to use in the kitchen and become further inspired and pleased with the *FoodWisdomRx* program. More determined than ever to stick with it to achieve wellness, we affirm the significance of remaining committed to the enhancing lifestyle changes we've already made and become, to an even greater extent, confirmed believers in the miracle of healing foods.

Life Lesson #40: *Healing from any disease, regardless of what doctors say, requires diligent effort, self-education, and action.*

We join excellent discussions and informative presentations, attend vespers and several other worship services, and I have the opportunity to confide in a preacher who sagely advises:

"Sometimes what we initially view as catastrophe is actually a blessing."

His statement pairs perfectly with the words I uttered at the first meeting with my oncologist, *"I'm going to come out of this better than ever and be able to help other people . . ."* I interpret this as confirmation that I'm listening to my God-Voice and doing as I'm being directed.

"All that we are is the result of what we have thought," the reverend says, quoting Buddhist philosophy. "The mind is everything. What we think, we become."

This reaffirms the information I received from the ice crystals.

Everything the cleric discusses supports what I've been doing all along.

These moments in the mountains prove miraculous, and I feel extraordinarily blessed as I continue to work at being positive in my conscious thoughts. I can only pray that my unconscious is receiving the messages.

Life Lesson #41: *All creation begins with thought. Be aware of your thoughts; work diligently to stay loving and positive.*

The minister smiles and suggests I sing *Every Little Cell in My Body is Happy and Well* to convince myself that I'm healed. "Sing it until you get sick of it to ensure the message is received internally!" he commands.

Melody, rhythm, and repetition impact the emotional center of my brain, allowing the transfer of important messages to my molecules and subconscious. Singing soothes me and helps me release dark emotions.

Through repetitive songs, I'm able to release the *fight or flight* instinct and relax into acceptance and relief. The 'happy cell song' is sung to the tune of Stephen Foster's *Shortnin' Bread* from the early 1900s, and I'm told that Wally Amos penned the lyrics.

I sing these profound words repeatedly day and night. Sometimes Barbara sings it with me and sometimes David. I imagine I sing this little ditty in my sleep. I desperately want my cells to get the message—and do you know what? It works!

Later, I discover that Unity Church uses the song to help with health issues. I rejoice in the miracle that it was presented to me and how it continues to give me comfort. Even when smothered by the darkness of the diagnosis, I never give up; I do everything in my power to become disease-free.

It's a beautiful, dedicated weekend during which I become even more aware of the miraculous pattern that persists: all that I need continues to arrive on the scene!

We make new friends and acquire new recipes while developing skills to improve our kitchen experiences.

I'm even more blessed because I receive confirmation of God-Voice directives: Think positive thoughts; work to remain clear and balanced; nature is instrumental in the healing process; and I must work at being well.

I *release my fears* and *thank God for the diagnosis* during silent prayer at a church service on Sunday, our last morning in Virginia.

An incredible sense of peace comes over me and has remained ever since.

I now look for blessings in every aspect of life.

Life Lesson #42: *Look to your trials and troubles; recognize their lessons so you may gain knowledge from them and rejoice.*

I become cognizant that when it's my time to go, I'll be prepared, and all will be as intended.

However, I am primed to continue my journey of evolution and revelation.

Warrior-Woman is going to prove the doctors wrong!

All of the resistance I had before relinquishing the fear vanished. Acceptance becomes the gateway to freeing my body, mind, and soul for healing through Love.

Life Lesson #43: *Give up your fears to God, to Source, and your burden will be carried.*

Life Lesson #44: *Accept your state of affairs so that the universe may unfold perfectly to reveal peace, freedom, and joy.*

As I perform this transformative work, I engage in an energetic shift of consciousness on a cellular level.

There is synchronicity in everything—every experience is shifting my cellular structure.

On the philosophical level, shifting consciousness opens space for my body to heal and supports the other work I'm doing.

I'm being transformed on a cellular level.

Loving myself becomes a catalyst for more miracles!

ACT III

EMBRACING THE RICHNESS OF A LIFE-TRANSFORMED

SCENE 1
An Emergency Hospital Visit:
Letting Go Becomes Another Lesson in Placing Myself First

> "Don't worry, I'm fine.
> Distress in my gut, twinges in my brain, creaking in my bones, spasms in my back, fire in my eyes. I'm fine—and dandy, too! Don't worry!"
> ~ JIMMI-ANN

*H*ealing my immune system and preparing my body with the right foods before chemotherapy is undeniably the best thing I could have done.

Thank goodness I needed surgery that afforded me eight weeks of healing time to do the work to get well.

Thank goodness the horrible side effects I imagined never materialized.

The chemo continues and I feel okay but exhausted most of the time.

I discuss my condition with the oncologist every third Tuesday when blood is drawn.

When I return to his office on Thursdays, if the bloodwork is reported satisfactory, I'm deemed healthy enough to take the next infusion immediately. Each session with the meds takes about half an hour longer than the one before because each dose becomes more potent. The first session lasts from one o'clock until five-thirty p.m. This is another reason art supplies and entertainment elements serve as helpful props.

The Second Chemotherapy Infusion: The doctor discusses my bloodwork after the first drip, stating that all tests come back *perfect*.

What an exhilarating update!

I believe the excellent news is due to a combination of prayer, my support system, attitude, foods, supplements, exercise, and medicine. However, after receiving a second *perfect* bloodwork report, David and I became further convinced that right-food is medicine.

From my journal, late August 2005: *Doc says the first chemo is always the hardest, and since I feel decent and have had very little adverse reaction to the medicines, I'm going to come through this with flying colors! Hooray!*

In contrast, the oncologist never said anything encouraging about my situation. It must be dreadful to work with terminal patients whom you ultimately lose. Doctors are apparently forced to go with worst-case scenarios—probably due to the threat of lawsuits and their own mental health concerns.

Doc is pleased that I feel good, look good, and am happy.

I tell him that I thanked God for the diagnosis and explain that I wouldn't be where I am spiritually, physically, or emotionally right now were it not for *the* cancer.

He's thunderstruck, although he'd prayed with us previously.

I tell him I've let go of my fears.

"If people could let go of their fear, they'd have a better survival rate," he continues, *"I am very proud of you and your determination."*

I seize those words and cling tightly to them—my God-Voice interpreting them as hope.

I am where I'm supposed to be, doing what I'm meant to do, and life is unfolding just as it was destined to evolve.

All. Will. Be. Well.

ACT III SCENE 1

The Third Chemotherapy Infusion: The third drip lasts from one o'clock until six-thirty p.m. Before contracting cancer, I had no idea that chemotherapy sessions are so lengthy. Perhaps it's an element of treatment not often voiced so that others won't feel uncomfortable. Still, I'm determined to share my experience to help make it easier for others facing a similar situation. Remember, initially, I was told there was no hope, but I stubbornly refused to believe it. I am so fortunate that I did.

To my surprise, the oncological facility offers their patients cookies, chocolates, peppermints, soft drinks, and all manner of sugary treats to help them get through chemo. Roxanne advised me to take "legal" snacks and beverages to my appointments, stating that Western medicine generally does not encourage good nutrition as a protocol for cancer patients.[12]

Impressed with my progress, the physician asked me the difference between conventional and organic foods. I'm surprised by his question, but I proceed to educate him to the best of my ability.

Recent research has revealed that today, on average, most U.S. medical schools require less than twenty contact hours of nutrition instruction. Based on my experience with the disease, this fact is horrifying!

Sad to see cancer fighters ingesting sugar to make them feel better during infusions, I begin to take alternative snacks to share. *Again, sugar is a cancer feeder, and cutting off sugar removes a crucial food supply to cancerous cells.*

From my journal, September 2005: At home . . . *The pills are no major problem. My eyes still burn when I become emotional, tears well up, and the pain remains intense, but I am learning how to control my feelings! The burning dissipates after about ten days.*

There's been no nausea or diarrhea. The cold still affects my fingers and throat, which has intensified because I'm not drinking enough water. All of this contributes to the development of calluses on my hands and feet that are aggravating, but I've been informed this is a common problem with chemo.

Hey, I know I'm lucky! Things are going exceptionally well with the meds!

Suffice it to say that Warrior-Woman is getting a little too cocky about the brilliant and brave way she's handling chemotherapy.

I take the third drip on a Thursday and forget to mention that my bowels have not moved since Tuesday. After all, what's a day or two?

Well, Friday rolls around, and nothing.

Barbara brings over some tea called "Smooth Move," which promises to help. But it doesn't, and I'm miserable.

My stomach is swollen and tight on Saturday, and I keep sipping the tea.

David brings me every item he can find from the pharmacy to help me achieve relief. Nothing works.

The tea, though tasty, still isn't helping.

Do you remember Life Lesson #23? *Don't be afraid to advocate for yourself?* Well, let's just say that I fall back into an old, ingrained pattern because I honestly don't want to bother the doctor over the weekend.

I'm not about to contact Roxanne for fear of recrimination; I *know* I've made a poor choice not to share my predicament with a professional.

Not smart.

Life Lesson #45: *You're only human; if you fall into non-productive patterns, accept them, rectify them, and challenge yourself to become more aware.*

I. Am. In. A. Mess. Of. My. Own. Design.

You'd think I would have finally learned to practice what I preach since I discussed the importance of placing oneself first to thrive, live life more fully, and be more available for others. But oh no, not this week.

ACT III SCENE 1

Much as I'd like to blame *chemo brain*, I know that hubris is the culprit.

My tragic flaw is pride.

Bullheadedness comes very close to thrusting me into a dangerous, life-threatening medical nightmare.

On Sunday morning, I'm determined to wait until Monday to call my oncologist. I'm still drinking tea, hopeful for movement.

Barbara is frustrated.

David is very frustrated.

I am more frustrated and obstinate than I've ever been in my life.

I keep drinking tea, eternally hopeful . . . then I vomit throughout the night.

Monday finally arrives. I'm beginning the seventh day of blockage. I insist David go to work.

I call the doctor's office, and his receptionist insists that I speak to Doc personally. He is not happy. He reminds me that I've been instructed to call him if I experience constipation or diarrhea.

I state meekly that I wanted him to have a good weekend.

There's a very pregnant pause . . . I can almost see steam coming out of the telephone.

"I'll meet you at the hospital—I'll have you checked in so you may go directly to your room," says Doc before hanging up abruptly.

Oh, dear.

I call Barbara, who agrees to drive me to the Cancer Center.

I manage to dress and have another cup of "moving" tea before her arrival. The tea makes me throw up.

I'm dry-heaving in the living room when she walks in.

The retching proves contagious—"Lucy and Ethel" try unsuccessfully to terminate spontaneous gagging, which, in turn, produces uncontrollable laughter and tears.

Gagging, laughing, and crying simultaneously, in this situation, is wretchedly painfull. On top of everything else, crying triggers the burning behind my eyes and produces a piercing headache.

Barbara absolutely *cannot* be around someone who is throwing up, and now we have a major problem. She grabs a bucket and dumps me in her passenger seat with the vessel between my knees—just in case.

With the radio playing loud enough to break the sound barrier, she rolls down her window and sticks her head outside as she drives so she can't hear me as I gag for fifty miles.

I am utterly exhausted when we arrive at the hospital; we're met like royalty and rushed to a private room.

At this point, I'm a 'retching ruin!

Two nurses get me into a hospital gown as I, a total wreck, collapse on the edge of the bed and wait . . . and *wait* . . . in dubious anticipation for *soon-to-arrive* Enema. However, before she arrives:

I feel . . . *funny* . . . in a peculiar kind of way . . .

There is a movement . . . It's smooooooooth . . .

"Outta my way!"

I dash to the bathroom and *almost* manage to close the door . . . almost.

ALMOST.

I *ALMOST* made it.

I almost made it.

Almost.

Barbara manages to escape into the hall—almost in time.

I am mortified.

They keep me overnight to rehydrate me and make sure things continue to move *smoothly*.

I'm "re-liquified" through an I-V that keeps me returning to the "scene of the crime" every twenty minutes or so. I think it's probably the most expensive bowel movement in the history of humankind.

God bless the nurses who remain consistently and cheerfully proud of me.

Of—*course*—they were.

Thank goodness Doc isn't present for the main event! He arrives

ACT III SCENE 1

after things settle down and gives me a well-deserved lecture.

He reveals that I'd been in a very dangerous situation. He's adamant that this must never happen again. It's vital that poisonous toxins be released from my body, and I'd stubbornly refused to ask for his help. Doc reiterates that self-care is my responsibility and that we barely avoided a debilitating crisis:

"Your colon has recently healed from surgery; if there had been a weak spot, your colon could have burst, and you could have died from sepsis."

Oh. My. Gosh.

None of us had considered that.

There could have been deadly consequences for my refusal to change my mind.

The episode ends well, but I'm incredibly lucky.

God isn't finished with me yet.

I'd felt virtuous, believing I was in command of my journey, but the hospital incident made it perfectly clear who is really in control. Though I'd given up my fears and thanked Him for the diagnosis, I still smugly believed that *I* was the one directing my destiny.

This experience becomes another revelation: Although I have free will, God is my ultimate director.

My self-judgment worked against me when I continued to make myself "right" or "wrong." As much as I endeavor to be non-judgmental of others, I now realize that sometimes I persist in judging myself. Becoming more aware of this limitation, I work at letting it go. Let God. He is the Master. I vow to do everything possible to stay on the path to complete His plan.

The hospital incident serves as a compelling reminder to be wary of ego.

Looking back, why did I not listen to my loving caregivers, the ones who hold my welfare paramount?

Unreasonable? Inflexible? Pigheaded?

Oh, yes, that's me!

Life Lesson #46: Never cling to a decision because you are stubborn; review the facts and change your mind if the situation warrants.

Life Lesson #47: Listen to and have faith in those who love you and advise you wisely.

Life Lesson #48: Self-care is crucial; it is neither noble nor loving to ignore your own needs.

Life Lesson #49: Hubris will triumph. Pride comes before the fall. Unthinking, poor choices inevitably come back to bite you in the backside!

Barbara, dear Barbara, remains steadfast as she elevates sisterhood to a whole new level.

I return home, trash the tea, and vow never to drink it again. I just wish it had moved me quite a bit earlier . . . or that I had moved my body just a little bit faster!

From my journal: *I am finally home after an overnight stay at the hospital. I'd become dehydrated; a lack of liquids exacerbated the pain in my hands and feet. The chemo-drip and inadequate water consumption prompted a gripping experience with constipation.*

My food coach says that people often have problems with hydration during autumn because of changes in seasonal energy, which also played a part in my distress.

Chemo dried out my system, and I went seven days without a movement. I was miserable and vomiting on Sunday night.

Doc sent me to the Cancer Center at the hospital on Monday morning, and, ultimately, I purged the 'mother lode.'

Or, as David says: "She hit a three-point seven on the 'Rectum Scale.'"

SCENE 2

Overjoyed! I Get My Kid Fix!
Teaching One Class Each Week Recharges My Spirit

"Hip, hip, hooray! Hip, hip, hooray!! Hip, hip, hooray!!! Welcome back, 'Miss' Jimmi-Ann! We missed you!"
~ CAMPERDOWN STUDENTS AT 'TODAY'S HOORAY'S' ASSEMBLY

Over the moon! Victorious! Exultant!
   Triumphantly, I strategize a way to further use the *stepping out* and *distractive action* tools from my Warrior's arsenal! My incision is healed by late August, and I'm determined to return to school to get my "kid fix!"

I return to Camperdown in mid-September to team-teach our weekly Multiple Intelligence class (MI.) This course, a transition-into-high-school program developed for our oldest group, is comprised of eighth graders. It meets on Thursdays, and our innovative curriculum offers the perfect opportunity for me to return home to one of my creative passions. I can design lectures and teach the class one day each week!

I can handle the hour drive into Greenville, impart knowledge, and drive an hour home. I believe this will benefit my state of mind, and my oncologist agrees.

Teaching and having contact with the unique energy of my students and colleagues provides a big boost to my spirit.

Our small, non-profit school operates like a family, and I did not like being separated from them. This morning class gives me time to return for chemotherapy on the days I'm scheduled to receive infusions. Driving for two hours back and forth to one weekly class will increase my fatigue, but I'm coming home!

Our headmaster routinely field-tripped small groups of students to visit with me over the summer. During these visits, students shared cheerful anecdotes, warm wishes, and crafty bits they'd created for me. The school also routinely forwarded homemade cards and artwork, and even long-lost former students I hadn't seen for years appeared to offer tender support.

Although delighted with their loving, uplifting energies—and feeling them all as joyful blessings—I want to be part of the action again. I need to see their glowing faces regularly and impart knowledge to their marvelous minds. I'm jubilant about returning to school; the decision is therapeutic.

Several co-workers comment that they've missed my laughter echoing through the halls, and we all breathe easier knowing I'm back in the building.

Our graduating class traditionally produces a Thanksgiving feast for homecoming on the Wednesday before the holiday. On the days before the feast, we hold a giving ceremony involving everyone in the school. Participants write words of praise and thanksgiving about a partner and present this gift of words aloud to the person whose name they have secretly drawn.

I introduced the practice in 1991 to help build confidence in writing and public speaking. I always take pleasure in this giving custom, but I am incredibly moved this year when I receive numerous offerings instead of the traditional single recognition. The beautiful declarations are further examples of how this school feeds my spirit.

This group prepares much of the food for the feast in crock pots and microwaves, then serves students, alums, current and former Camperdown families, and staff.

As the director and designer, I'd always relied on a warrior-like character to make it through the hectic preparations! This year, I have to pass off the leadership of the feast production and—instead of working myself to the point of exhaustion moving furniture, props, and decorations while helping aspiring cooks prepare and put finishing touches on the dishes—I adjust to simply enjoying myself and having fun.

David enjoys a reprieve, too, since I always used to kidnap him to help with the festivities. The feast, inside a massive tent on the soccer field, proves to be a great success, and I'm moved beyond words by the appreciation and warmth expressed by what seems like multitudes of well-wishers.

Life Lesson #50: Compliments are often thought of but not articulated. Never hesitate to compliment others, for compliments are priceless.

Reconnecting with students and faculty proves rejuvenating!
I try to arrive early on MI Thursdays to visit with students before classes and catch up with news I've missed—and it's almost as if I've never been away.

Life Lesson #51: When you want something, go for it—you are capable of turning desires into reality if you put forth the effort.

The idea of Multiple Intelligences, introduced in the 1980s by Harvard developmental psychology professor Howard Granger, centers around the belief that people are smart in areas not measured by Intelligence Quotient (IQ) tests. The IQ assessment measures verbal-linguistic, logical-mathematical, and visual-spatial abilities along with testing speed. Granger identifies interpersonal, intrapersonal, naturalist, musical, bodily-kinesthetic, and existential intelligences as other ways people may be smart.

The Thursday after Thanksgiving, when teaching interpersonal intelligence (people smart), I ask the class to come up with three adverbs that express a positive way of feeling "fine." Students agree on *fantastically, magnificently,* and *wonderfully*. We also discuss how expressing oneself in approving terms can affect others favorably. I'm setting the stage for our next unit, intrapersonal intelligence (self-smart), where we traditionally introduce positive self-talk, a lesson it's taken me a lifetime to learn.

During an assembly the following year, I relay that when asked how they feel, people most often respond *fine*, whether their mood is terrific or miserable. Why not have a more imaginative answer than *fine?* I ask.

As a school, we resolve to use the three adverbs to express our feelings. Our response: *fantastically, magnificently, wonderfully fine!* becomes the standard.

After the school adopted this positive phrase, everyone reported feeling fabulous, and the expression continued to be used for years and years!

Do you know what? If you say it, you begin to feel it! It demonstrates one of the weapons Warrior-Woman employs to fight Cancer: *Say it until it becomes true.*

If you try the feelings phrase in public, you may well be surprised at the response!

Many people say I 'make their day' when they ask me how I feel and I give them such an unexpected answer. I love to watch their expressions, and frequently, after I explain its history, they decide to begin using the same response as well!

"Do it," I tell them. "You'll feel better for it, as will the receiver!"

Life Lesson #52: *Spreading light and love is infectious. Encouraging others to smile improves your own outlook.*

SCENE 3

My Warrior's Arsenal Proves Victorious:
Happy Halloween, Happier Thanksgiving, Happiest Christmas Ever!

"Bliss feels like this!"
~ JIMMI-ANN

We feel abundantly blessed as we approach the holiday season with Hope and Anticipation.
Chemotherapy continues, and I keep myself well-hydrated!
Warrior-Woman, cloaked in loving possibility, rejoices in the splendor of living.

From my journal, late September 2005: At home . . . When I go in for a CT scan on Friday to see if there's been any progress with shrinking the tumors, I'm in a room with other patients waiting for radiology tests. I begin testifying and cheerleading for organic foods, supplements, and exercise—typical Jimmi-Ann.

Suddenly, as I approach the CT machine, I'm overwhelmed by Fear and "What Ifs." My apprehension been under control since I thanked God for the diagnosis, so I'm surprised at my transient reaction. However, I remind myself that to have misgivings is only human. I get over

STAGE 4 TO CENTER STAGE!

it after a good cry. Fortunately, I'm two-and-a-half weeks off the chemo drip, and my tears do not cause me pain.

At the doctor's office—early October 2005: After going in for bloodwork on Tuesday, David accompanies me back to the office on Thursday to learn the doctor's evaluation of the various tests and the scan. The bloodwork comes back "perfect"—again!

Doc shows us the CT pictures on his computer. Placing the July CT and October CT side by side for comparison, he points to four small tumors on the July scan and notes they're missing from the one in October! The middle-sized tumor is nearly gone, and the golf ball-sized tumor is now thirty percent smaller.

Doc advises me to keep doing what I'm doing because it's working!

David and he are so delighted, I think they may begin to dance! Instead, I grab them both for a giant hug, and they hug me back!

I'm scheduled for three more rounds of chemo starting Thursday before another CT to see what's happening inside my body.

I feel deeply in my heart that Christmas is going to be especially merry this year!

With my mind, body, and soul in great shape, I'm overjoyed to still be on this planet!

Life Lesson #53: *There are no words to describe the absolute bliss felt when hard work shows indisputable results.*

At the doctor's office, Halloween 2005: I show up dressed as Johnny Depp's Mad Hatter from *Alice in Wonderland*. I am delighted that almost everyone has joined the holiday spirit with festive costumes and props. As I enter his office to discuss the results of Tuesday's blood tests, Doc is studying his computer.

"Perfect bloodwork again," he reports as he swivels his chair around slowly, takes off his glasses, and twirls them.

ACT III SCENE 3

He grins.

I smile.

"I believe you just might beat this thing!" he says, looking me square in the eye.

Again, it's as if all sound stops, all movement ceases, and the world stands still as his words sink in.

Overcome with joy, my tears flow . . .

Doc smiles broadly—I can tell he's just about as overwhelmed with this incredible news as I am! "Jimmi, you have a big responsibility to help others by sharing your process."

"Oh, mercy, I've realized this from the get-go and primarily communicate my experience with curious cancer patients by word-of-mouth and referred phone calls. I've tried from the beginning to get everyone I know, or even chance to meet, to understand what I'm doing and how it's working—even though, early on, I didn't completely understand it myself."

"Good for you—get the word out there! And keep up the hard work!"

"Yes, sir."

"Since your therapy comes in a six-pack, you'll have two more infusions after today," He continues, "It's too early to look see if it's gone, but we'll run another CT scan after the sixth chemo treatment."

I receive the fourth infusion that same day and feel okay. My reaction to the drugs remains the same.

So very blessed and so very grateful; Barbara and I are *both* delighted that I've retained my full head of hair!

Ninety-eight chemo pills for two weeks cost twenty dollars with my insurance co-pay. Without insurance, they would have cost $1,678.95. The six times I purchased them would have cost more than ten thousand dollars without *the* cancer policy. What a miraculous God-Incidence that I'd purchased cancer insurance through the school! Extreme gratitude.

I believe all of this will be over in six weeks!

But no matter what, I'm in an incredible place spiritually, emotionally, and physically, and overjoyed to be alive.

Life Lesson #54: *Suffering is an invitation to self-love, self-recognition, and self-healing.*

Even though I'd obtained an excellent cancer policy, receiving benefits becomes a nightmare. It takes over five months of emails, telephone calls, and handwritten letters to get my settlement on track. Exhausted, I have to work several hours a day trying to get satisfaction from the insurance provider.

For the first time in our marriage, we find ourselves heavily in credit card debt because of such incredibly slow bureaucracy. Mounting interest on the debt is not, of course, covered by the policy. It's disgusting that it takes all this effort and energy—energy I could channel instead into improving my health—to finally be awarded the settlement that's rightfully mine. Cognizant of our financial distress due to the insurance company's incompetence, Barbara insists on gifting me the *FoodWisdomRx* program. Incredible . . . but that's Barbara!

From my Journal, November 2005: *I received a fifth infusion, which resulted in similar reactions to the chemicals.*

Doc and the nurses make more eye contact with me than ever—they even smile at me. Now I realize why they initially seemed so aloof. How devastating it must be for their souls to work daily with the terminally ill! My heart goes out to these brave caregivers.

The day after my fifth infusion, David announces that we're going out for breakfast the following morning and leaving the house at five a.m. Though exceedingly odd, I know the morning repast is his favorite meal, so I'm all in. I'll take my legal food, and he can splurge on pancakes if he desires.

"Dress very warmly, wear your boots," David tells me. "And don't forget your gloves. Also, dress in lots and lots of layers."

He's incredibly considerate of my severe reaction to cold winter temperatures due to the chemotherapy, and he takes exquisitely exceptional care of me.

We leave when it's still dark, and as we approach our destination, he misses the turn, mumbles something, keeps driving, and pulls the car into a field.

Suddenly, we're surrounded by a clutch of cousins! They surprise me with my first hot-air balloon flight, courtesy of the owner and pilot—my cousin Anthony! I feel like a super-cared-for three-year-old as David stuffs me into a snowsuit, and I waddle toward the balloon.

As I'm lifted into the basket, Anthony directs my husband and grins, "Jump in, David! You're coming too." Surprised and thrilled, David vaults over the side.

Greeted reverently by a spectacular sunrise while drifting in the peaceful morning breeze, immersed in tenderness and affectionate gestures, this magical escapade is one of many unique experiences I'm presented during my journey.

I'm very appreciative to be so very well thought of and marvel at the astounding amount of love that continues to intensify!

Thanksgiving 2005: Sixty-three family members gather to share blessings, laughter, and food at an extended family gathering at our eldest daughter's home on Thanksgiving.

We are overwhelmed with gratitude because so much of the food adheres to my food plan as the family shows their thoughtful, compassionate support in such a considerate manner. Our loved ones have become more food-conscious due to my experience. David's weight loss and improved health due to the consumption of clean foods also inspires them.

Happily, healing with food is now a family tradition.

From my Journal, December 17, 2005: *I visited my oncologist on Tuesday and reported the usual sensitivities. Doc listens to me gravely, then asks:*

"You do know this week's injection may be your last, right?"

"No, sir!" I gasp as my jaw drops. "I would have remembered if you'd told me that."

When he'd said that I'd finish the six-pack and complete a few tests, I assumed that more treatments would follow. Now, as he tells me this could be the last dose based on the progress I've been making, I'm stunned.

Only six months ago, we were told that, statistically speaking, I would be dead by now without treatment—that I'd be on chemotherapy until I die!

My vow to take only one six-pack of the drug has become a reality!

I feel as if I'm floating, awash in joy and boundless thankfulness, that the impossible yielded to the possible!

Warrior-Woman's courage to wage war on Cancer results in another triumph!

When I go in for another CT scan on December 12—the day my mother passed away fourteen years ago—and then return to the doctor on December 19 for his interpretation, I believe that she will help bring wonderful news about my most recent scan.

We're also ecstatic about Barbara, who, after six months on the plan, has found that five of her issues are now non-existent—and a sixth is vastly improved. Feeling like her old self again, she believes her transformation represents undeniable proof of miracles and that our new lifestyle is the key to wholeness and health.

From my Journal, December 19, 2005: *My bloodwork again scores a "perfect" at my oncologist's today, and I believe now more than ever*

ACT III SCENE 3

that I've never experienced dreadfully severe reactions to chemotherapy due to the food plan, exercise, my positive attitude, and everything I've done to fight Cancer. But there are still some shadows in my liver, and Doc—who's become progressively more positive about my case—wants to see them more clearly as he believes they may be dead cancer cells.

However, he decides to stop the therapy now that my six treatments are over. He ordered a PET scan for Monday, December 26, hoping it will reveal more clearly how my liver is functioning.

I remain in positive spirits and continue to act as if what I desire has already happened!

Christmas 2005: We stayed overnight Saturday, Christmas Eve, with our "matchmaker daughter," my former student Deborah, and her family. When she was in high school, she introduced me to her dad, and we fell in love at first sight. Incredibly intuitive, Deborah told us later that she knew we'd marry if we ever met. She chose me as sweetheart for her father and has become the daughter of my heart; she made me a grandmother! My life is so incredibly blessed! Thank you, Deborah, for our God-Incident marriage!

Inseparable since we met, loving and laughing our way through life ever since, David and I witness the special gift of three grandchildren's excitement over a visit from Santa. Having lost last Christmas to the virus makes this day even sweeter.

Later, as we drive home, I proclaim: "It's a wonderful life, and I couldn't possibly be any happier!"

December 26, the day after Christmas: The PET scan is scheduled at the hospital after lunch on Monday, and David accompanies me for the critical assessment. We've promised to notify Barbara immediately as soon as we know anything.

The PET scan,[13] which uses radioactive tracers injected into my bloodstream to see what's going on in my entire body, requires me to remain motionless in a recliner, in the dark, for ninety minutes as the radioactive material moves through me, assessing every system and organ.

I use the time to sing *Every Little Cell in My Body is Happy* softly to myself as I visualize my ecstatic reaction due to impeccable health!

I'm tired afterward, but fatigue is my new normal.

We sing Christmas carols on the way home, filled with high expectations for another "perfect" report from the doctor at my next appointment.

We arrive home to see our answering machine light flashing red.

"Doc doesn't want you to have to wait until the nineteenth for the news!" his nurse practitioner declares excitedly. "There's no evidence of cancer in your liver and no evidence of bone lesions! There are no living cancer cells *anywhere* in your body!"

Our joyful noises are most likely echoing throughout all time and space!

Thank you, Jesus! Thank you, Guardian Angels! Thank you, Mother and Daddy!—Their two marvelous souls are undoubtedly dancing in heaven, reveling along with us!

We can now attest that it's possible to be even happier than I was on Christmas day! Experiencing this magnitude of perfect ecstasy, I stand firm in my belief that true richness is *life*!

I'm really and truly alive—consciously living every glorious new day. My timeline is met. I am pronounced cancer-free!

WE DID IT!

Merry, Merry Christmas!

BELIEVE!

We laugh, jump with thankfulness, dance with glee, and shriek with gladness!

After we calm down just a little, David, with his irrepressible wit, proclaims: "I couldn't be happier if you'd given birth to twin millionaires!"

SCENE 4

A Strong, Powerful New Me:
Angered by a Third Surgeon, I Invent the Cancer Patch!

*"Ninety-nine percent of the
world's population are idiots..."*
~ GARY

" . . . we all take our turn."
~ DAVID

Exultation! Buoyancy! Freedom!
"No drawing of blood today!" says Doc.
He's almost as happy as David and the conquering Warrior-Woman—who is about to burst with happiness!
As we meet with him to discuss his interpretation of the PET scan, chemotherapy is a thing of the past!
Doc reiterates that my unique story must be shared, and I'm thrilled when he tells us that he's looking into nutrition options for his patients!
"The scan shows absolutely no live cancer cells anywhere in your body," he continues. "However, dead tumors are lingering in the liver and mustn't remain there." He scheduled an assessment appointment for me with a surgeon for early February.

"I'm impressed and grateful for all your hard work," he tells me as he shakes my hand and continues, "Your surgeon will schedule an MRI to guide him during surgery."

Doc embraces me, and then he and David exchange a hearty man-hug.

I ask him about the itchy port before I leave.

"Have it removed," he laughs. "No use inviting the cancer back!"

The same former student's doctor father removes the port he'd inserted, sterilizes it, bags it, and hands it to me.

I look at him, dumbfounded.

Bewildered!

He laughs and says, "Knowing you, you'll turn it into a piece of jewelry!"

(I haven't . . . at least not yet.)

Boldly, Warrior-Woman again seizes the spotlight, this time to take action against the dreaded antagonist, Surgery.

I don't want to be cut! I don't want another operation!! I fashion posters stating: *The tumors are gone—no reason for surgery. MRI baffles doctors. Physician, heal thyself. YOU are the physician! YOU ARE the physician!* I place these computer-generated posters around our home to remind me to act as if what I desire has already happened.

David and I meet the new surgeon on a Monday morning, and he schedules an MRI for three days later to determine the intricacies of removing the dead cells.

"You know, doctor," I say, "I received exactly what I prayed for—no more chemo and no more cancer! Since the last PET scan, I've been focusing on praying the tumors away."

He stares at me, sneering as he replies: "If prayer worked, I wouldn't have a job."

I'm shocked speechless by a physician *again!*

I keep hitting the jackpot with surgeons—what a churlish lout!

Livid, I hear him say something about me returning the following

ACT III SCENE 4

Monday when he'll explain the MRI and schedule surgery, and the receptionist hands us an appointment card.

"That man is not laying a hand on me," I fume as we stride toward the car.

"You got that right," David agrees as we both slam our car doors dramatically.

"He can believe whatever he wants but has no business saying that to a patient."

"Yes, ma'am."

"I'm so mad I could . . . I could . . . I don't know *what* I could do!"

"Go ahead."

Silence . . . .

"You know what?"

"What?"

"I'm going in on Thursday to get that screening. We'll come back on Monday to hear the results. Then we'll abscond with the MRI and find another surgeon."

"Great plan!"

"And you know what else?"

"Tell me."

"I'm going to go home and make a cancer patch!"

"Oh yeah?"

"You've heard of a nicotine patch? I'm going to make myself a cancer patch!"

"OK . . ."

"I'm going to be like those vessels of water in Japan, and my words are going to make that doctor understand that prayer works!"

David grins and starts the car . . . .

I do it! I make a postage-stamp-sized *faith sticker* that I place over my heart. I wear it constantly. I even sleep with it on. I put up several large posters around the house, repeating the same message: *Tumors are gone. No need for surgery.* Armed with my newly embraced self-compassion, I'm determined to make that doctor eat his words.

When I wake up Thursday morning, it's snowing!

Snow! Glorious snow!

This was before technology deprived us of inclement weather days—when we teachers wished for snow far more fervently than students. Mental health days are always a blessing! In fact, today is the *single* bad weather day that shut down businesses and schools during the 2006 school year. Even though I'm not scheduled to teach because of the medical procedure, I rejoice with my colleagues because it's *snowing!*

I receive a call from the hospital—the radiology department is also closed due to hazardous weather conditions. My MRI is rescheduled for Saturday morning, giving me two more days for the patch to do its work!

I take great pleasure in my day—I chat with Barbara on the phone, take a walk, play with Buzz in the snow, and make a big pot of fresh vegetable soup and a cake of gluten-free cornbread. In my heart, I know this will somehow lead to another God-Incident.

Magnetic resonance imaging (MRI) is a non-invasive way for a doctor to evaluate the organs, skeleton, tissues, and all bodily systems with 3-D images that can be viewed from all angles.[14] The MRI machine used to evaluate my liver is long and cylindrical. The tube is basically a giant magnet that realigns water molecules in the body with radio waves long enough to take internal pictures in cross-sections of the body.

On Saturday morning, I drive to Spartanburg, remove the patch for the first time, lay without moving in the coffin-like tube, complete the scan, put the patch back over my heart, and drive home.

I'm still wearing the patch as David and I return to the surgeon's office and are escorted into an examination room Monday morning, where we wait . . . and wait . . . and wait.

ACT III SCENE 4

Eventually, an intern enters and apologizes, saying the surgeon has been called away for an emergency and cannot see us.

He reports: "The MRI revealed no tumors, only a benign cyst that doesn't need to be removed, and you don't require surgery."

Warrior-Woman and David make eye contact and laugh triumphantly.

The patch worked!

Miracles happen, but you have to make the effort and truly believe!

Doctors might get more vacation time if more people follow a path of self-appreciation, hard work, positivity, and belief in miracles!

The Warrior is gloriously victorious again!

As we exit the room, another door opens, and the surgeon steps into the hall. He looks at us, startled; I guess his *emergency* has been resolved.

"I-I-I'm pleased you don't need surgery," he stutters as we peer at him.

I smile, "Prayer works."

SCENE 5

Another *FoodWisdomRx*™ Experience: *An Adventure in Fasting to Encourage Post-Chemo Toxin Elimination*

> "May your guardian angels keep you safe . . .
> on the right road . . . and outta trouble!"
> ~ DAVID AND JIM

Roxanne suggests that her clients fast several times a year to rest overworked organs and eliminate toxins. She supervises these fasts with group and private phone calls, which evolve, over time, into Zoom meetings. Barbara and I are advised to join her mid-January cleanse. I know I'll benefit particularly from eliminating toxic metals to which I've been exposed during chemo, MRIs, and scans.

Even though we don't like the idea of going without food, we understand the rationale and decide to give it a try to rest our organs and trash our trash. The *FoodWisdomRx* fast includes rotating food remedies: tiny portions of broths, soups, and special salads. Vitamins, supplements, cleansing teas, and lots of water are also essential to the experience.

We pack our bags, coolers, and supplies. Fleeing from our husbands is vital because we'll probably climb walls and try to eat furniture.

ACT III SCENE 5

A friend loans us her beach house on the sound in Charleston, and "Lucy and Ethel" are poised to embark upon another road trip! David and Jim laughingly call on angels to accompany us, knowing our antics often result in *interesting* situations.

We laugh with our loves, kiss them goodbye, and hit the road—eager to create new memories. We're both finally "back to normal"—if you could ever say that about either one of us—and we head delightedly toward the coast. Luckily, our incessant babble doesn't divert us, and we drive straight to our temporary home base.

We plan to enjoy our five days—assuming we don't starve to death first!

Our senses are on full alert, and we drink in the magnificence of the coast, which is gorgeous!

After rapidly unloading the car, we nest, then pull out our fasting instructions to study. There's lots of preparation for concocting remedies.

We begin with the *sweet veggie broth* recipe, an insulin regulator good for softening tightness caused by heavy food consumption that relaxes the body. We gather the required assortment of vegetables and merrily dice, slice, and chop them. After dumping the cabbage, onion, carrots, and butternut squash into a gallon of water, there are more remedies to prepare, and we begin—then the doorbell rings.

Cautiously, curiously, we approach the front entrance . . .

Rosie is standing on the veranda, grinning!

Surprise! Hallelujah! Yippee!

Our 'guardian angel' has arrived to help us!

Fearful that "Lucy and Ethel's" shenanigans might lead to a *fast-disaster*, the sisters have gifted us a seasoned helper for assistance and encouragement!

After lots of giggling and hugs, Rosie notices that our vegetables have started to boil. She reduces the heat to simmer. Again, cooking vegetables at low temperatures extracts nutrients; we will eventually strain the bulk and drink the broth.

STAGE 4 TO CENTER STAGE!

We help her unload and unpack and then exchange stories while she directs us into the kitchen, where we continue to prepare more remedies. We acknowledge our pleasure as she teaches us more cooking tricks.

We become bosom buddies forever.

One of the remedies calls for garlic, and Rosie asks us to peel several bulbs. Barbara and I eye each other as our noses twitch, and we do our darnedest to peel those diminutive bits with our fingernails.

"Let me show you," Rosie says suddenly as she chuckles with amusement. She takes a clove from Barbara, places it on a cutting board, and says: "Look, take the flat of your knife, place it over the clove, and smack it with the heel of your hand." She removes the blade, picks up the garlic, and peels the papery skin from the bulb.

Intrigued, the incompetent *sous cooks* grin—as you may surmise, this skill is utterly foreign to both of us but easy and enjoyable once we understand the process. We have a grand old time, releasing our frustration every time we whack the garlic bulbs with our knives. Peeling garlic turns out to be surprisingly therapeutic! As Rosie demonstrates how to chop, mince, and slice it, we vow never to purchase prepared garlic again.

We make remedies that can be assembled and stored in the refrigerator for a week, and then Rosie sets us to work creating another favorite recipe. Waldorf salad, Roxanne style, for our dinner as she grills a beautiful, fresh white fish she purchased from a local fish market. We sit with our now traditional twig tea, overlooking the sound, enjoying a delightful final meal together.

Our carefully planned and presented not-eating adventure begins bright and early the following morning. Adjusting to the first day is simple because we're on a strict schedule with instructions for taking vitamins and supplements, drinking water and specific teas, and consuming remedies. We enjoy ourselves, although we're a bit uncomfortable due to hunger.

Day two becomes easier . . . so far, no furniture eating or wall climbing! We're blessed with Rosie's presence, enthusiasm, instruction, and companionship.

We learn that the first two days of abstinence calms the body, and we're already beginning to feel much lighter. Our sleep has deepened noticeably in only one night!

Wow, abstaining from food isn't so bad!

We are told we'll experience clarity and significant energy increases on days three through five. Amazingly, we can see our stomachs shrinking! Astonished that we feel so buoyant, boundless, and free, Barbara and I wonder: *If eating very little makes us feel so extra-ordinarily wonderful, why eat?*

Oh, dear.

There I go with an unwise thought about my well-being and self-care.

Barbara says she feels the same—liberated, free-floating, and light.

Colors are more brilliant, sounds clearer, and our sight sharper; we are amazed at how great we feel.

Despite experiencing mindboggling euphoria now that I've permitted my organs to rest after working non-stop for fifty-two years, I'd never stop eating!

Roxanne shares a list of possible side effects. She tells us to call her if uncharacteristic aching, stiffness, headache, stomach issues, or other unusual symptoms occur so she can adjust our food intake and advise us on different food remedies for individual cases. Ignoring symptoms can be dangerous.

Energized by how wonderful we feel, Barbara and I are glad Rosie's right in there with us. We're like three giddy playmates enjoying exploring the region while basking in the charm of each other's company. And we experience pleasant downtime, taking naps, reading books, and journaling.

I receive another perfectly delightful surprise when Barbara presents me with a whimsical shadow box she created at home, emblazoned with David's pronouncement after our prayers had been answered: *I couldn't be happier if you had given birth to twin millionaires!*

We share laughter over Barb's imaginative representation of my husband's words. I cherish the delightful little box that symbolizes both David's declaration and the unwavering nurturing of my two champions. The memories it generates every time I gaze at it never fail to produce a smile.

Our interlude in Charleston proves to be a magical time and another God-Incidence for which I give thanks.

The recurring pattern persists: *Everything I need keeps revealing itself.* And I'm amazed at its precision!

Life keeps proving more incredible than I'd ever expected it could be.

My improved self-esteem set me free. As I now see the world through eyes of self-acceptance and compassion, my perceptions change—I discover clarity of thought and become more consciously aware of *everything*—especially the countless miracles that are mine for the taking. I am overjoyed to be chock-full of life!

Life Lesson #55: *Liberate yourself with divine love to better embrace the miracle of being alive!*

Day three dawns beautifully.

We become even lighter, and our sight sharper as the day progresses.

We adhere to our cleansing schedule, but my joints begin to stiffen by evening, and I sense the shadow of a headache.

I call Roxanne to ask if I should change my protocol.

She questions me but gives me the okay to continue. If my symptoms worsen, I should make a puree with adzuki beans and eat it with the gluten-free crackers we have in case of a toxin elimination overload.

I don't want to eat and ruin my progress, and I'm okay except for the stiffness.

Although my joints become more rigid near bedtime, I don't mention it to my cohorts; I figure a good night's sleep will fix everything. Besides, I've dropped six pounds in three days and love it! This means I've lost one hundred and twelve pounds since the initial virus a year ago!

Elation! Exuberance! Ecstasy!

I'm over the moon!

Morning dawns bright and beautiful, but disaster strikes as I'm cock-eyed with pain! I'm so stiff I can't get out of bed, and my skull feels like it's about to explode! I try desperately to lift my head from the pillow, but my whole body feels as if a giant magnet is holding me immobile. Rising is impossible.

Terrified, I shout for my friends to help me.

Immediately comprehending the situation, Rosie races off to concoct a puree and grab some crackers.

Barbara hauls me into a sitting position.

She doesn't have to say a word, for I can read her thoughts: *Oops! You did it again.*

I'm disappointed, embarrassed, and annoyed with myself.

You'd think my previous hospital episode would have taught me the importance of self-care, right?

I told you I'm stubborn—and perhaps I am selectively forgetful, too!

Rosie dashes in with the food remedy, and after a few bites, I can feel my muscles begin to loosen, and the stiffness and headache begin to dispel.

I finish eating, and then, as my mobility returns, I *shoo* my friends from the room and get dressed.

Later, when I enter the kitchen, Rosie is on the phone. She hands it to me, saying: "Roxanne wants to talk to you."

Oh, dear.

Roxanne explained that the heavy metal toxins from the chemotherapy had lodged in my joints and muscles, and the proper food remedy moved some of it through my body. The liver functions as a filter for the body, and eating adzuki hummus loosens trapped poisons in that organ.

I haven't ruined my fast by eating food not on the plan, and the difficulty I was having assures her that even though I did everything right in conquering Cancer, I was heavily burdened with chemical toxins.

If the symptoms return, I should call her without hesitation. She advised me to get a lymphatic massage that afternoon if I could arrange it because that would help open the flow of the lymphatic system to dump the toxins from my body.

Even though I've raised my consciousness concerning health care, I'm still teasing an old pattern: *I hope things will improve—let's wait and see what happens.* An epiphany crystallizes: this was the mindset I embraced when I dragged an aching leg around for nine years before discovering I needed hip replacement surgery!

Wow! When I get stuck in a pattern of thought, it tends to hang around for a long while! Ceasing this way of thinking is challenging, but now, at long last, I've red-flagged my thought process after suffering through sufficient examples of what happens without continued awareness—and luck! From now on, I endeavor to become more mindful of this tendency and be truthful with myself by avoiding the creation of scenarios about what I *hope* will happen when I am in distress.

Life Lesson #56: *Hope is best served with commitment and action rather than imaginings.*

ACT III SCENE 5

Good fortune resumes as I connect with a massage therapist who sees me that afternoon. I almost dissolve under her masterful manipulations, and as she works, I can feel movement in the areas where my lymphatic system flows smoothly again.

Barbara and Rosie shop and play tourist while I'm on the table for two hours.

Rosie eases me back on the fasting regimen sweetly and thoughtfully, producing the scheduled vitamins, water, and tea I missed while on the table. We head back to the house for remedy time as a quarter cup of aged miso soup with wakame beckons!

Limp as a dishrag. I drink extra water to push those nasty toxins from my system and then luxuriate in an exquisite, warm Epsom salt bath, which makes me feel fabulously nurtured and peaceful. I'm in paradise!

Some of Roxanne's other clients are cleansing for the entire week, but as "first-timers," she recommends we break our fast with a light dinner on the fifth day. We help Rosie prepare a feast of small portions of butternut squash soup, seafood, fish, salad, and chocolate mousse. Our taste buds sing in appreciation as we celebrate victory and the new, treasured memories this adventure has provided.

After sleeping deeply, we share a "Roxie and Rosie" breakfast before preparing for an early morning departure and heading home. Grateful for the experience, we decide to make fasting a permanent part of our health regimen. We now recognize the value of resting our organs and ridding our bodies of poisons that inevitably find their way inside.

We've experienced a glorious, illuminating five days, but perhaps, best of all, Rosie gifts each of us with servings of chocolate mousse for the road!

ACT IV

THE CURTAIN CLOSES BEFORE RE-OPENING TO SPECTACULAR EVER-NEW BEGINNINGS

SCENE 1

Hello, Dolly!— Living in Bliss— *Before the Parade Passes By!*

"Life is a spectacular,
awe-inspiring rollercoaster ride!"
~ JIMMI-ANN

Our twelve, graduating, eighth-graders take what they've learned in Multiple Intelligence classes and transform into teachers at an all-day Learning Fair in the spring. Each student, with the help of a mentor teacher, plans three levels of lessons, rehearses, and teaches six classes on Learning Fair Friday. It's a fantastic day of student-led scholarship; we catch a glimpse of the adults these young people will someday become.

A co-worker, Meg Coffey, passes me in the hallway after I've just taught my Thursday class the day before the fair. She says, "Hello, darlin'."

"Hello, Darlin'," I reply.

"No!" she corrects me. "I said, 'Hello, Dolly!'"

I must have looked baffled because she laughs and explains: "The Greenville Theater is holding auditions for 'Hello, Dolly!' soon. You should audition. You *are* Dolly Levi!"

"Yeah, right."

"Think about it," she advises as she walks off, then turns, gestures grandly, and says: "Hello, Dolly."

Ridiculous! As a teacher, I don't have the time or energy to engage in acting—at least not since 1984 when I performed in the musical *Stop the World I Want to Get Off*. Having withdrawn from performing to direct students in plays instead, it's been years since I've auditioned for a show.

Oh my. Now I have the time and the energy. Though cancer-free, I've taken a full year sabbatical due to the dreadful diagnosis, and my scholars are in the care of a charming, inventive, inspiring young colleague as I continue to teach my MI class and work with special projects. Then again, a theater professor at university had once stated that I majored in leading roles.

Might I *be* Dolly? After all, musicals are my passion . . . *No! No way! Forget about it . . .*

The following day, Learning Fair Friday, I return to school to see the eighth graders' stellar performances as teachers. (A humorous side note: At our debriefing after the fair, we seasoned educators chuckle when one of our youthful student-teachers inevitably says: "I had no idea teaching is so exhausting.")

Twice during the fair, Meg and I pass in the hall and twice Meg grins and shouts: "Hello, Dolly!" She's called me Dolly three times now, including yesterday's greeting!

Suddenly, I freeze, stunned.

I look toward heaven and exclaim: "Okay, God, I get it!"

He's placed yet another miracle in my path. I'm going to play Dolly Levi!

As noted, one of my deep-rooted patterns is that it generally takes me three times to *get* something. Remember? Two health scares, and I did nothing to remedy my collapsed immune system. It took a deadly ailment to get me off my backside to fix things. Now, it isn't merely Meg's words—her three reminders are another God-Incident! I'm gifted another opportunity to follow my heart and possibly share my life's passion—after David, of course.

ACT IV SCENE 1

Life Lesson #57: *Don't talk yourself out of doing something that feeds your spirit, especially with excuses that come automatically.*

I must remember that Miracles are always present; all I need to do is pay attention. I've learned how crucial it is to slow down long enough to grasp what is mine for the taking!

I get to work and begin to research the role. I purchase the soundtrack, learn Dolly's songs, and relentlessly envision myself as Dolly. I think like Dolly, walk like Dolly, develop Dolly's attitude.

I study the non-musical version of Thornton Wilder's play, *The Matchmaker,* analyze Shirley Booth in the old black and white film, and watch Barbara Streisand in the role. I live and breathe Dolly Levi. I'd never approached a character with such intensity and preparation using Warrior-Woman's device: say it until it becomes fact!

Never a true method actor until I "became" Dolly, I stride determinedly into auditions *as Dolly Levi.* It's *Dolly Levi* who glides to the piano when it's her turn to sing and calculatingly blows them away with her rendition of the title song.

Dance auditions go well—I nailed it!

Asked to return for callbacks, I know God has led me to this most extraordinary opportunity, and, in my heart, I *know* I'm Dolly Levi before it's announced the following night at the theater.

Thank all of Heaven!

Thank you, and God bless you, Meg!

Look out, Broadway!

Although I experienced a devastating blow nearly a year ago, I still, somehow, assume the powerful role of warrior and am able to delve deeply to discover exceptional Faith and arrive at this totally unexpected and astonishing place in my life!

The cast enjoys seven weeks of rehearsals, and we become a close-knit family, which often occurs when imaginations merge in the creative process to give life to a theatrical event.

It feels magical to be working in live theater with a marvelous company that genuinely respects and supports each other. We live, laugh, and are each other's universe during practices and performances.

Sometimes Barbara accompanies me to rehearsal, as does David—to enjoy the energy of artistic inventiveness and to see me removed from cancer worries and thriving in splendidness. *I couldn't have been happier if I had given birth to . . . well, you know . . .*

My walks become dual-purposed as I work lines and rehearse while hustling down country lanes. Preparing songs during my walks is cathartic; sometimes, neighborhood dogs join in concert. I continue my six a.m. swims. I rehearse Dolly's entrance and sing the title song as I 'float down the stairs into Harmonia Gardens' every time I descend the YMCA's multiple steps from its entrance. I sing, dance, and act to my heart's content.

I'm genuinely delighted with every aspect of living and oh so very thankful to be alive.

Hello, Dolly! holds a preview performance to a packed house and receives a standing ovation one year after *the* cancer diagnosis.

The next day, the morning of our opening, I bend over to pick up a piece of paper, and my artificial hip pulls out of joint!

Down I go like a bag of wet cement!

I manage to pull the phone off the nightstand. David's at work, so I call Barbara, and she and Jim break into our house to rescue me.

They call EMS, and off I go to the emergency room in an ambulance that seems to lack shock absorbers. The ride is so horribly jarring that I heartily shout each time we hit a bump, "Thank you, Jesus! I feel the pain!"

The EMTs look at me strangely, having no idea why I'm grateful for pain.

I am feeling pain because I'm *alive!*

I am deliriously happy to be alive!

An orthopedist assesses the situation in the emergency room.

ACT IV SCENE 1

He believes I crossed my knees as I retrieved the paper, instigating disaster and making my leg temporarily unstable. They're about to set my hip when the doctor notes that I'll be in too much pain to perform tonight.

Poor man, he has *no idea* with whom he is dealing!

Warrior-Woman: "We're opening that show at eight o'clock tonight, come hell or high water! A little joint problem is not stopping me! Not now! Not after all I've been through! Give me as little morphine as possible so its after-effects won't hinder my performance! Let's get this show on the road!"

My friend just shakes her head and smiles.

After wrenching the apparatus back into its normal position, I'm placed in a temporary cast, ensuring my stability.

David arrives, worried but relieved after a discussion with the doctor. I'm so very fortunate he appreciates living with craziness.

Nothing is stopping me now!

Barbara calls my director. He wants to postpone the opening, but I won't hear of it.

My two angels get me to the theater by 6:30, and I'm in costume and makeup by quarter after seven.

Several local newspaper reporters are allowed a brief interview. A capsule of my story will hit tomorrow's papers, and the account will be covered in depth the following week.

The cast is informed they'll have to adjust to my situation for opening.

The curtain rises as scheduled!

Dolly likely made musical theater history that performance—almost certainly the only one ever to be wheeled around the stage by her choreographer in an 1890s wicker wheelchair!

Our dance designer, dressed as a nurse in period costume, appeared to be an essential element of the show if one didn't know the situation. She pushes me to my appropriate marks at the correct times since she knows all my blocking and dances—and I remain in that chair for three performances, acting, singing, and "dancing" from my essence!

We play to full houses and stellar reviews.

News of *Dolly* being wheelchair-bound spreads like wildfire. After the first performance, we welcome numerous audience members in wheelchairs—and it's a humbling experience.

Actors at this theater traditionally hold a backstage meet and greet after the show. I was stunned when fans in wheelchairs gushed:

"Thank you so much! You were in a wheelchair, but I forgot about that—maybe I can act too! I really want to act—now I'm going to go for it! My disability has kept me from auditioning, not anymore! After seeing your performance tonight, I might have the courage to audition! Maybe I can be an actor too! Thank you!"

These remarks elevate me to unimaginable levels of bliss!

Miracles are ubiquitous once we become mindful—once we truly believe!

That night, I became a glorious God-Incident myself!

Never-ending blessedness!

Last week, I wasn't allowed costume changes because my leg had to remain immobile. This week, I'm back on both feet, a triumph over adversity, continuing to prove that the show—and most especially that my *life*—must go on! I'm thrilled to be changing my wardrobe and getting back to Dolly's extravagant sense of style.

Numerous current and former students and their families attended the show. Intimates I haven't seen in decades from high school, college, and even *Lost Colony* friends show up to see me as Dolly. Family members and well-wishers attend performances to witness my determination to wage war and the testimony to how much I want to live.

David attends all fourteen performances, and Barbara is there for most of them. However, she focuses on watching David as he watches me during one show. She witnesses the overwhelming love and pride radiating from his soul; so much emotion is pouring from him that her own spirit feels blessed.

Every night at the end of Act One, I have the unbelievable prophetic good fortune to sing *Before the Parade Passes By*. I weep with joy each night, singing lyrics about regaining vitality, embracing purpose, pursuing dreams, and genuinely living. Every word in that song has significant meaning to me, as it illuminates my incredible soul journey and self-awakening.

God gifted me a most exquisitely perfect moment in time and a most exquisitely perfect song to showcase my astonishing rebirth.

I am humbled.

I am abundantly rich.

Rich with life.

Rich with love.

Rich with family.

Rich with friends.

Positivity, extraordinary Faith, Strength, and Determination brought me to physical wellness, mental acuity, and a spiritual evolution I'm still learning to navigate.

All the way from *Stage 4 to Center Stage!*, I have been re-gifted with precious life.

Life Lesson #58: *Awaken to the reality that true richness is the gift of life itself!*

The husband of another dear friend with whom I'd taught for many years hugs me after a performance and whispers, "Why the hell are you teaching school?"

His words make me smile, but encouraging young people to be curious and creative, helping to build their self-confidence, and imparting life skills to them are other genuine passions for which I have bubbling enthusiasm.

Before cancer, I considered myself a jack-of-all-trades and a master of none. It took facing Death and self-realization to understand that I'm truly the master of many gifts. Finally, at long last, I understand that believing, being grateful for, and utilizing my talents is a responsibility I must accept to continue developing my character as God directs.

My two earthly guardian angels beam from the audience. It's almost impossible to believe that we've gone from agonizing despair to phenomenal bliss in one year. We'd probably have difficulty believing it if we hadn't lived it.

With new-found confidence and belief in myself, I set out to conquer my adversaries, achieved that goal, and have been blessed with more than I could ever have imagined!

Warrior-Woman has always been an aspect of my character; she was always waiting in the wings to spring forth upon command. However, she can relax now because Jimmi-Ann is on the path she was born to traverse. I am blessed beyond words and grateful for every breath I take.

I am alive.

I am aware.

I am *amazing*.

I *am* a miracle.

Life Lesson #59: *Never doubt that miracles occur.*

Life Lesson #60: *We are ALL miracles placed on this planet to love.*

Every performance closed with a standing ovation.

My feet never touch the ground.

I am delivered to a place I never knew existed, where I float and soar. I ride wave after wave of benevolence, beauty, and an indescribable tenderness that permeates my being. I am grateful to be *more* alive than I ever imagined possible; I want very much for my story to inspire others to discover their own path to living life more fully.

Knowing that the closing of the show will prove a resounding blow to the natural high I'm riding, Roxanne throws a closing night cast party unlike any before! She conceives of "legal" party foods that range from surprising to exotic and afford mouthwatering nutrition for every palate!

Barbara creates fantastic decorations to glorify the celebration further and perfumes the setting with countless flowers.

The cast, crew, guests, and I are all enchanted.

And when Roxanne stashes extra chocolate mousse cups for us to take home—remembering "Lucy and Ethel's" enthusiasm for mousse indulgence—it's definitely a magnificent climax to an incredible year!

Wiser, stronger, and ever-so-much richer for the experience, I've evolved—now I *live* and *breathe consciously*, delighted and thankful for every new day.

The curtain has fallen, and I excitedly embark upon the next exciting act of my *continuing* life drama!

Life Lesson #61: *If one person can achieve the seemingly impossible, every single one of us is in the position to do the same. We are far more likely to realize our heart's desire if we truly believe in possibility.*

SCENE 2
How I Have Changed:
Several Years Later . . .

"Life is a joyous adventure once we truly accept
and appreciate the effects of God's love."
~ JIMMI-ANN

*I*t occurs to me after *Hello, Dolly!* closes that I'd been in so much pain before my hip replacement that I'd given up singing. Melodies that were once a daily blessing vanished, and I hadn't sung for nearly twenty years! Blessedly, music is restored to my life by the cleric at the retreat, in hospital waiting rooms, and with the musical. Now, I continue to sing, as singing makes me happy!

Coincidence?

No.

God-Incidence.

I discussed cell-memory earlier in the book. For several years after winning the war with Cancer, I became depressed in May and even more so in early June. Eventually, I identified a connection between the unwanted emotions and the disease. My depression coincided with the occasions of the original colonoscopy and the Stage 4 diagnosis.

I finally realized that cell-*memory* was returning me to troubled thoughts. Once I became conscious that my fears were due to my *cells remembering the* cancer, I was able to dismiss the anxiety.

ACT IV SCENE 2

Dealing with resurging emotions was fairly easy, and when I acknowledged them, they disappeared. Once I reminded my cells that I am *happy and well*, this particular memory, buried deeply in every cell, was erased. I no longer find myself despondent during spring and summer!

Before the illness, I spent many hours reading because I took great pleasure in learning new things and traveling vicariously through the written word. These days, I find that I don't want to miss anything. I still enjoy reading but pay more attention to experiencing real life—*in the now*!

Biker-Babe and Biker-Dude hit the highway to take to the road in anticipation of adventure!

"I want to go on a motorcycle ride!" I announce after I'm declared healthy, astonishing David.

He nearly has me institutionalized, thinking I've lost my mind. David rode motorcycles in his youth, and I asked him to stay away from them before we married because they frightened me. He agreed readily since he hadn't ridden one for years anyway.

"Guess what I did?" he laughs two weeks later. "I bought a motorcycle!"

Gold Wings are very large bikes, so riding is not as scary as I'd imagined.

He begins wearing Hawaiian shirts in protest of leather (even though we both have leather gear for cold weather.) I make him a bandana with a ponytail attached to wear under his helmet to compliment his 'costume.'

I become a queen on my throne, riding behind him, having fabulous adventures, and *living*.

Blue skies and tailwinds!

One day, David mentions he's always wanted to learn to fly.

Having learned from my illness to stop putting things off, it's time to expand our horizons even further!

We train as pilots and learn to operate an airplane!

We prefer flying together, and I'm overjoyed to co-pilot as we take to the skies and experience delightful adventures up in the air and in places we discover through our travels!

It's difficult for me to grasp that I've piloted a plane *alone* and landed *safely!*—more than once, just another example of living my life to its fullest.

Wild-Woman gets to laugh and scream to her heart's content!

David abhors rollercoasters while I'm bonkers for them, so when he surprises me with an adventurous rollercoaster holiday tour where I can ride, laugh, and scream like the crazy lady I am, I'm all in!

During this trip, he insisted on loyally escorting me on multiple rides despite personal aversion, another demonstration of his unwavering affection.

A fabulous frolic in the deep blue sea!

During a different trip—to Florida—I was ecstatic to swim with dolphins—something I dreamed about but never considered making a reality until Cancer taught me to live life more authentically. Frolicking with dolphins is magical, and I'm so very grateful to be *consciously alive* to experience the marvels of this beautiful planet!

Life Lesson #62: *Live life to its fullest; make time for adventure and joy.*

Surprise! Surprise! Surprise! An astonishing birthday surprise!

Wendy Coburn, a beloved, delightfully feisty student I taught in the 1980s, throws me a surprise birthday celebration at Anita's Mexican restaurant. More than twenty former students, most of whom I directed in high school musicals, are in attendance, as well as our children and grandchildren. We're so fortunate that Wendy has remained a constant and vital part of our lives, and we both treasure her in our hearts!

ACT IV SCENE 2

I am incredulous that these former students showed up to express their fondness and gratitude for the impact I have made in their lives. I haven't seen or been in contact with most of them for more than twenty-five years! Wendy presents me with a perfect blessing; I am forever thankful!

The restaurant staff, who took such good care of me when I was undergoing chemotherapy and who we regard as family, joined the celebration as well. It is a most fantastic birthday! I remain, for all time, moved beyond expression.

God continues to reveal the influence of my actions on the lives of others, and every positive deed, expression, and kindness returns tenfold in unexpected deliveries.

It's a miracle when we finally understand how every little kindness, random smile, or *God bless you* in response to a sneeze can positively influence another—and possibly even save a life.

For me, the stimulating process of teaching, creating, and being with eager young people is essential, so I revive the role of full-time teacher! I appreciate the challenge Camperdown Academy provides, enjoy working with my colleagues, and treasure educating my students.

I also delight in mentoring Tiffany Depuy, who took over my classes during my sabbatical and uplifted young scholars in my stead. We complement each other beautifully and find great excitement and fulfillment in inspiring children to act, dance, create art, participate in theater combat, and help design and build costumes, sets, props, and tend to publicity for the six or seven productions we produce annually.

Our seventh graders traditionally study and perform *Romeo and Juliet* in preparation for ninth-grade English class. As dyslexics, making friends with Shakespeare in middle school sets them up for success as they further their education. Their involvement with and understanding of Elizabethan history and lifestyles helps them internalize the bard's words. Tiffany's contribution as assistant director and choreographer enhances every aspect of the show, especially the ballroom scene, with her wonderful and surprising approach to Renaissance dance. Her clever and innovative ideas inspire me; our collaborations are terrific.

Often, I write plays to channel my passion for writing and ensure that my actors are assigned the perfect character to develop self-confidence and foster success. Other than plays, we have quite a hectic schedule as our department provides opportunities for students to develop life skills through art production and shows, a Renaissance Festival, a Haunted House, Thanksgiving Homecoming, a Christmas pageant, a lip-sync concert, a joke show, Laughter Yoga—and the list continues.

Of course, there's the instruction, too. It's wonderful to be back in the classroom full-time!

I wrote an outline of this book soon after my recovery, but life took over, and I didn't make time to resume the development of a full-length manuscript. Although I've written several scenes, it will sit in an inert state on a shelf until inspiration strikes—waiting until I instinctively know the moment is right when I can complete it.

Meanwhile, I'm blessed to share my account as a motivational speaker and have made lasting relationships through these conversations. I remain available for—and to talk with—patients seeking encouragement to fight the horrific illness.

Roxanne sometimes refers clients to me for motivation, and I take great pleasure in encouraging and supporting them.

My story so moved Amelia Aiken that she embraced *FoodWisdomRx* wholeheartedly. David and I, Amelia and her husband, have become the greatest of friends. Recently celebrating her sixth year of being cancer-free, Amelia and Jim are both enthusiastic followers of the program. He has dramatically improved his health and well-being; Jim suffered from an eye condition that was leading to blindness—*right-eating* corrected what was baffling his medical doctors. Miracles abound!

Breast cancer runs in Barbara's family, so when she's diagnosed with Stage 2, she immediately armors herself for war. Embracing Positivity and Determination, my champion fights and wins her battle and has remained free from the sickness for ten years. Fortunately, Doubt and Fear did not plague her because of the many possibilities and opportunities my experience revealed during the extraordinary journey we shared.

I'm very thankful she could handle the disease more easily by employing what she learned. Thrilled to be her inspiration, we joyfully appreciate and embrace our countless blessings together!

Sometimes, I stand outside, lift my arms to the sky, and say, "Thank you!"

David and I are so very blessed and happy for our continuing time together. We acknowledge life and love as precious and treasure each new day. The two of us now live *consciously* and with *intention* because we learned the hard way that every single moment is a gift. Our faces sometimes hurt because we smile so much—isn't that wonderful?

We are thankful for the joy, easiness, and contentment inherent in our ever-growing Oneness.

Our lives just get better and better.

Sometimes, I am overcome with positive, loving emotion because I am alive! I am love. I am loved. I am.

SCENE 3

Blesséd Exultation
The Magic of Being Love!

"Life became a magical journey once I cast off Fear and grasped the importance of living in the present while loving myself."
~ JIMMI-ANN

I am more convinced than ever that true richness is the gift of life itself.

It's now eighteen delightful years since I was declared disease-free, and I am forevermore grateful.

It takes a worldwide pandemic to create space in my life to continue producing this manuscript. When I began writing this time, it became challenging to do anything else because the flow has been incredible. David encourages me to stop sometimes because I need to move or eat since I sit and write for hours.

At least I generated something productive during shutdown!

Once my creative juices emerge, I don't want to sever imaginative thought. A realization crystallizes during this period: I'm so hyper-focused on the artistic procedure that I don't make time for other things—a *carryover* from my busy teaching/directing life! Thankfully, I've learned that self-awareness is half the battle for any challenge I encounter. I'm now mindful that better self-control in the creative arena will serve me well.

I've dreaded the unknown and change for as long as I can remember, and the pandemic forces me to rethink possibilities. As a drama teacher, I can't imagine teaching with communication restrictions because I believe that nearly ninety percent of communication is non-verbal, and a high percentage of that is through facial messaging.

I choose not to return to teaching in 2020 and ask instead to stay on the school's books for a year, thinking I'll return after the virus is under control. I'm informed that faces will be covered in 2021 as the school year begins. I've been teaching for forty-one years and decided to officially join David on permanent vacation.

"It's time to rewire and re-fire; I'm tired enough; I'm not going to double the tiredness by re-tiring!" Amenie asserts.

Terrific suggestion!

Nevertheless, I'm still apprehensive as I abandon my *living in the present* philosophy for a bit and agonize about leaving my profession. I fall into an old pattern as I fail to apply one of my lessons and project my negative, worrisome, imagined scenarios about abandoning the workforce.

Although my fear of the unknown, life-after-work miasma, proves unwarranted, I realize I've learned many, many lessons during the war with Cancer—and in the ensuing years. Employing them all consistently can be exceedingly difficult. However, I choose to step into the theater of the unfamiliar while appreciating that these stumbling blocks are valuable learning experiences, and life continues even more gloriously.

Although *the* cancer story climaxed eighteen years ago, the saga of my life miraculously continues. When I chose Love over Fear by utilizing all the modalities that were presented to me, with determination and hard work I was able to vanquish the dreaded disease! I remain a thankful student, cheerfully learning every day. Each morning brings new opportunities to give, share, and, most significantly—to *love*.

Finally, I'm able to treasure the marvel that is Jimmi-Ann. I am a walking miracle and a very appreciative one!

Loving myself is the greatest gift and the most incredible legacy. This message lies at the foundation of everything else I've discovered because I rejected my worthiness for such a long time. Early in my evolution, I abolished destructive self-talk. Self-love allowed me the freedom to sing, dance, laugh, and rejoice during the crisis when a more common reaction might have been to feel sorry for myself.

Employing positivity, I chose to *live* rather than dwell on the horrible prognosis and surrender to Death. What I discovered under my self-inflicted doubts, worries, and fears is more blessedness than I can comprehend. In loving and knowing my true self, I'm able to understand and value others to an extent never before possible. I am joyfully blessed just *Being*!

Each of us has a responsibility to attend to mind, body, and soul. I've always been cognizant of the need for balance. Nevertheless, I procrastinated, troubled with secret beliefs that I was inadequate and unworthy. That death sentence forced me into action.

A whole new world was revealed when I focused on loving myself and avoiding negativity! Joy and opportunity became boundless. Life is a fascinating, magical journey, and I eagerly anticipate each glorious new day.

David and I continue to delight in surprising our grandchildren, from riding motorcycles to piloting airplanes to swimming with dolphins! What adventure will we embark upon next?

A flying machine! A flying machine!

David decides to build an experimental aircraft that we can land in our field. I traveled with him to Mexico, Missouri, to take airplane building classes.

Yep, I take on the role of Rosie the Riveter, although he does most of the work. He becomes lost in his creativity, and I take enormous pleasure in supporting him during this exciting venture.

An air-flight school in Lawrenceburg, Tennessee, teaches transitioning from a conventional plane to an experimental one. So, we load ELSA, *Experimental Light Sports Aircraft,* into a U-Haul and head for the Volunteer State! (The wings and tail are taken off the fuselage for transport.) Flying a short take-off and short-landing airplane is very different from the Cessna in which we trained.

These classes and flying prove both fun and very rewarding. We experience great times and acquire terrific new friends while making incredible memories in Tennessee.

I used Roxanne's carefully planned elimination menu exclusively that first year, then eventually began designing my own meals because I understand the model. David and I continue to meet with her via Zoom to stay on track, along with feedback from the face and feet pictures she analyzes. We've adhered to her program so well that we're great examples of what eating the right foods can do for you.

Eating to live is *not* a diet. It's a lifestyle choice to which we are dedicated. Eating clean food is fundamental to good health and well-being.

Renée Brigman's mother, Emilie, lived to be almost eighty-six (nearly eighteen years after her diagnosis of Stage 4 cancer). If you recall, Emilie's association with *FoodWisdomRx* became my second miraculous God-Incidence, and the following statement is the denouement of her chronicle. Here is the rest of her story, in Renée's words:

My Mom might have lived longer if she had been willing and able to maintain the no sugar/no additive lifestyle. About five years before she died on April 13, 2021, she began to make choices to include off-plan foods in her diet that she missed. As the cancer began to grow in her again, she gradually lost vitality, making it harder and harder for her to do what she needed to be doing. We knew she was eating off-plan on the side, and we didn't make an issue of it. It's always a personal choice; she knew the consequences.

I think the moral of her story (if there is any long-term moral) is important. Maintaining recovery (not sure about survival because none of us survive life in the end) depends on constancy and persistence. She did a great job for a very long time, and we are grateful for her extra time with us. Her hard work for all those years was a wonderful gift to us.

I doubt I'd be alive today had I never heard Emilie's story.

I am forever grateful for her inspiring cancer warrior's determination to conquer the disease and the motivation she was to me. Renée and I became friends, and I count her as a blessing far beyond the life-saving messenger role she played in the drama of my life. Emilie's story further illustrates the importance of making healthy food choices.

Very gratefully, David and I continue to adhere to the *FoodWisdomRx* plan. The produce department of the organic grocery store has become my pharmacy. Now in my seventies, I take no prescribed drugs. Instead, I've learned to use food as fuel and medicine—I no longer use food as emotional solace.

I understand the fundamental importance of moving my body, and I seriously doubt I would have survived Cancer without exercise, which provided sufficient oxygen to my cells to retard rapidly growing carcinoma. Yet "falling off the wagon" of the physical movement element of self-care has become a character flaw.

My excuses?

Too busy, too tired, too lazy, even *too creative*! (Does the hyper-focus of the creative process make exercise the victim of creative flow? *Of course, it does!*)

Now, back to exercise—when I become motivated to work out, I push and overdo it. Sore and stiff, I fall back on excuses, and it's easiest to do nothing. My lack of exercise has resulted in a twenty-pound weight gain.

I know from experience that three consecutive days of walking, even a relatively short distance, improves my stamina, agility, and attitude. After writing this narrative about the importance of self-care, I vow to practice what I preach and become more physically fit. I must get outside in nature to further improve my health and amplify my glow!

Five years ago, when I was tested for nearly everything under the sun because my other hip needed replacement, I experienced an *aha!* moment—realizing that my hip had become an excellent reason to have slacked off on exercise.

This time, I don't procrastinate—as soon as I recognize the symptoms, I make an appointment with an orthopedic surgeon to schedule surgery. I want to get the operation behind me as quickly as possible.

Interestingly, it takes close to four months for surgery to be approved. I wind up in a wheelchair—and in terrific pain—for nearly a month. Praise Jesus, I'm *alive* to feel it!

The surgeon runs test after test after test after test, fearful perhaps of my previous medical issues. Every single test keeps coming back *perfect*—my immune system remains in tip-top shape. Surgery is eventually scheduled. *I share this with you now to reaffirm the impact that eating right continues to have on my body.*

Barbara, ever loving and supportive, suggests I ask the orthopedist to pray for me before surgery and play music during the procedure. He acquiesces but says I should wait to give him my calming classical music preferences until I'm in the operating room because he'll likely forget.

Though slow to schedule my operation, this man is excellent and thorough—*finally*, I've retained an admirable surgeon!

David is with me as I await transfer to the operating room. I'm *feeling no pain* when one of the surgical nurses, a former student, enters the room grinning. Thirty-four years previously, I directed her as Daisy Mae in a high school production of *Li'l Abner*. We hug, giggle, and sing songs from the musical.

STAGE 4 TO CENTER STAGE!

They come to wheel me into surgery.

It's showtime!

Everything proceeds according to plan ... *almost.*

Later in the evening, the orthopedist joins us in my room. He is laughing, "Well, your *performance* during surgery was unlike anything I have ever experienced."

"My what?"

"Your performance."

"What do you mean?

"You didn't request your classical music."

"I didn't?"

"No. You most certainly did not," his laughter increases.

"Oh, mercy. What did I do?"

"You demanded Broadway show tunes!"

"I did?"

His eyes sparkle, "You *sang* during the entire procedure!"

I gasp.

Silence ensues ...

"Really? I *sang* while you were operating on me?"

"Yes!'

"I *sang* through surgery?"

"Yes! All the way through ...."

"You've got to be kidding!"

"The nurses who knew the lyrics sang with you! It was a stimulating two hours of entertainment!"

David chuckles with delight.

"You certainly re-defined 'operating theater' today!" my surgeon is still laughing.

"Lord, have mercy! I *sang* while you operated on me!"

I have no memory of anything after singing with my former student.

Zounds!

I *sang* all the way through surgery!

Amazing!!

When God gifts you, He goes all in!

Singing again after years of silence due to suffering was one thing, but to sing *during surgery* is frankly stupefying!

I am *living* proof that the ability of our bodies to heal is enhanced by hard work.

Affirmations stimulate a positive response from our very cells. I believe we can help manifest things we want through positive thinking and eliminating negativity as much as possible.

Live in the moment; I know this is easier said than done, but it's unbelievably freeing when one can do so!

Remember, when destructive thoughts come through, place them in a bubble and release them into the atmosphere, where they will travel to the far reaches of the universe, burst, and become meaningless.

Have faith and act as if your desires have already been granted.

I continue to embrace Faith, Hope, and Positivity as I navigate my life's journey.

Once more, having compassion for myself changed my very existence as it allows me to create my life in the present. My time is no longer consumed with worrying about a past that's over and done, nor do I entertain feelings of unworthiness.

I recognize and offer gratitude for my blessings. I anticipate each new day with childlike wonder: Life is magical! Life is full of delight!

Once I learned to recognize my value and ended the negative self-talk, I became powerful beyond imagination.

I now acknowledge and embrace the lessons life provides; if I falter, I forgive myself and continue to move forward.

Over time, I internalized fundamental teachings that were instrumental to my recovery, two vital lessons are: to release Fear by embracing self-confidence and to regard desires as already accomplished.

The release of Fear is essential to absolute self-love.

"There is no fear in love," John 4:18, King James Bible.

Fear is the *opposite* of love, not hate.

I was filled with fear when I didn't love myself completely. Love eclipsed fear when I acknowledged its possibilities! Once I embraced my own worthiness and stepped into love, my fears faded away! I became whole. I became the person I was born to be!

Life Lesson #64: *Fear and negativity cripple us, limit us, and keep us from becoming who we were always meant to be.*

Why is it that we rarely hear positive stories about people beating Cancer?

Why does the media choose to dwell on the negative instead of the profound?

Why would most sources be interested in my story only if a breakthrough drug was discovered?

It's a mystery—or is it?

We live in a culture programmed to believe that medicines are the best way to get through the day and that a little pill will cure everything.

Wake up, world!

God provided us with amazingly magnificent vessels capable of healing themselves. While medication is sometimes warranted, we have the responsibility to cherish and care for our bodies—to move them, strengthen them, rest them, and nourish them without causing harm.

We are literally killing ourselves through lack of self-care and with foods that have been genetically modified, bombarded with chemicals, enhanced with antibiotics, and supersized with hormones.

Look to the incredible vessel you've been gifted, and work to respect and honor it through your choices and actions.

Listen to your inner voice, your God-Voice; it is essential to who you are.

Strive to do what you know is right.

Try not to overthink.

Remember, from the book of Matthew, we can move mountains if we have faith as small as a mustard seed: I am living proof.

A challenging component of my journey was believing because society often teaches us not to believe, not to trust, not to love ourselves. Happily, I found the enduring faith to believe, to let go of worries, and to have compassion for myself.

Remember: *If one person can achieve the seemingly impossible, every one of us is capable of doing the same; if we genuinely believe in possibility, we are more likely to attain what we most desire.*

My discovery that changing the world starts internally initially surprised me, but it seems so obvious in retrospect. I had to stop, look inward, and listen, then use those discoveries for transformation.

Imagine how glorious the world would be if we *all* understood that self-love, self-belief, and caring for oneself would result in a peaceful, loving planet!

Release your heart and open your eyes during *size* life story!

Love yourself to free yourself.

Open your heart to the Miracles offered.

Remember, God didn't make rubbish. Who are you to be self-critical? *You* are His dazzlingly splendid handiwork!

Listen to Intuition, embrace Miracles, and embark on the most exciting venture of *Being*.

Empowered by the love of David, Barbara, and the multitude of characters who joined me for this most extraordinary enactment, helped make it possible for this Warrior-Woman to surge to victory. The supportive compassion gifted to me by family and friends remains awe-inspiring and humbling; I was lifted by their strength, love, and laughter as my faith and hope intensified. My thankfulness is never-ending.

Experiencing the journey from *Stage 4 To Center Stage!* began spontaneously, then took on a life of its own; I am forever transformed.

My life's drama continues to expand as a whole new existence is revealed. As I enter the playhouse with boundless Delight, Opportunity finds me poised for my next exciting adventure!

On the day of diagnosis, I vowed that I'd be enriched by the experience and that other people would benefit from it; I have seen that prophecy become a reality.

My wish is that this account becomes an inspiration for others' personal growth and loving evolution. We are *all* magnificent, spiritual *Beings* placed upon this planet to *love*.

My life continues to be rich and full, and I eagerly anticipate each grand and glorious new day!

I am so very blessed and so very grateful to be joyfully alive and loving every moment!

I would not change a single second!

Life Lesson #65: *Life is a great adventure—hold on with your heart and savor every instant with sweet appreciation!*

EPILOGUE

"Jimmi-Ann, you're always full of surprises and never cease to amaze me. Every day with you is different and surprising. Every morning when I wake up, I look over at you and think, 'I want to live this moment for the rest of my life."
~ DAVID

David A. Muse

I imagine that writing this book was much like giving birth and that these pages are the offspring of arduous labor. I can, of course, appreciate the amount of work that went into this production. We all affect our environment and the future in many ways. Although Jimmi-Ann and I never had children of our own, she has hundreds, if not thousands, of young minds that have been uplifted by the force of her considerable personality—as a schoolteacher and role model for her students.

I've witnessed firsthand how my own children, now grown, have been positively influenced by her, and they all love Jimmi-Ann unconditionally. I've been positively affected, too, and believe in the power she wields so effortlessly. I hope you, too, will come to love her words. I know in my heart that—even though she might not know each and every reader of this book—she loves you all just the same.

~ **Curtain** ~

APPENDIX A
Life Lessons: Stage 4 to Center Stage!
A Guide to Lessons Learned

*"I did not do this by myself.
Never-ending gratitude for divine intervention
and my extraordinary supporting
cast of angels on earth."*
~ JIMMI-ANN

Life Lesson #1: Life's journey of discovery is ever-changing and never-ending; it requires persistent attention and nourishment.

Life Lesson #2: Miracles happen continually; if we pay attention, we become aware of them.

Life Lesson #3: God wants us to ask for what we desire.

Life Lesson #4: We have the power to choose how we feel, so work to stay positive.

Life Lesson #5: Every day of your life is a gift and should be embraced with gratitude, love, hope, and joy.

Life Lesson #6: If we allow fear to be a motivating factor in our lives, then we never truly live.

Life Lesson #7: Perceived tragedy can evolve into the greatest of blessings.

Life Lesson #8: Embrace a loving and forgiving spirit; make every effort to be at ease and delight in the gift of life.

Life Lesson #9: Be careful what you ask for because God wants to provide!

Life Lesson #10: If you expect respect, it is essential to respect others!

Life Lesson #11: Express gratitude; never hesitate to appreciate and thank individuals who positively affect your life.

Life Lesson #12: Unconditional love is a most precious gift; acknowledging it is overwhelmingly sweet.

Life Lesson #13: Hopelessness is not a strategy; positivity is power.

Life Lesson #14: Trust that the unexpected can lead to amazing possibilities.

Life Lesson #15: Listen to your intuition, your God-Voice, and take action accordingly.

Life Lesson #16: Just because something is unusual or beyond your experience, give it a chance; it might be exactly what you need.

Life Lesson #17: Miracles come in many different guises; pay attention and accept them with loving gratitude.

Life Lesson #18: Clean organic foods are a pathway to wellness.

Life Lesson #19: Showing compassion is a matter of choice; becoming aware of the feelings of others helps us make kindhearted choices.

Life Lesson #20: If you have an incredible partner, express your appreciation frequently!

Life Lesson #21: Don't be afraid to try new things; you might just be pleased and surprised at the outcome.

Life Lesson #22: It is true that we are what we eat! We may use food to improve our health or hurt our bodies.

Life Lesson #23: Don't be afraid to advocate for yourself; most people will be happy to help if you are sincere and grateful.

Life Lesson #24: Positive thinking is essential in every aspect of our lives and will open doors to miracles if we remain optimistic.

Life Lesson #25: Stop putting off things you want to do; life is to enjoy now—this very day!

Life Lesson #26: Never doubt the effect you have made upon those whom you encounter.

Life Lesson #27: God is Love; He does not want us to suffer.

Life Lesson #28: You are unique in all the world; open your eyes and recognize your gifts; accept and use them gratefully.

APPENDIX A

Life Lesson #29: God is all-powerful; it is our soul responsibility to have faith.

Life Lesson #30: There are powerful dormant abilities within each of us waiting to be discovered; believing in and accessing these gifts is a birthright.

Life Lesson #31: God's gifts of self-love and self-acceptance become easier with daily practice.

Life Lesson #32: Strive to become a living example of God's love.

Life Lesson #33: The greatest gift of all is unconditional self-love and self-acceptance.

Life Lesson #34: Through love, miracles are manifested.

Life Lesson #35: Proper food *is* medicine.

Life Lesson #36: The human body is a miraculous instrument with the ability to cleanse and heal itself if treated as a holy vessel.

Life Lesson #37: Miracles are available for the asking and the believing; believing is the challenging part.

Life Lesson #38: The planet is glorious! Offer appreciation and gratitude for all of creation!

Life Lesson #39: Getting out in nature is comforting, calming, uplifting, and healing; make embracing nature a priority.

Life Lesson #40: Healing from any disease, regardless of what doctors say, requires diligent effort, self-education, and action.

Life Lesson #41: All creation begins with thought. Be aware of your thoughts; work diligently to stay loving and positive.

Life Lesson #42: Look to your trials and troubles; recognize their lessons so you may gain knowledge from them and rejoice.

Life Lesson #43: Give up your fears to God, to Source, and your burden will be carried.

Life Lesson #44: Accept your state of affairs so that the universe may unfold perfectly to reveal peace, freedom, and joy.

Life Lesson #45: You're only human; if you fall into non-productive patterns, accept them, rectify them, and challenge yourself to become more aware.

Life Lesson #46: Never cling to a decision because you are stubborn; review the facts and change your mind if the situation warrants.

Life Lesson #47: Listen to and have faith in those who love you and advise you wisely.

Life Lesson #48: Self-care is crucial; it is neither noble nor loving to ignore your own needs.

Life Lesson #49: Hubris will triumph. Pride comes before the fall. Unthinking, poor choices inevitably come back to bite you in the backside!

APPENDIX A

Life Lesson #50: *Compliments are often thought of but not articulated. Never hesitate to compliment others, for compliments are priceless.*

Life Lesson #51: *When you want something, go for it—you are capable of turning desires into reality if you put forth the effort.*

Life Lesson #52: *Spreading light and love is infectious. Encouraging others to smile improves your own outlook.*

Life Lesson #53: *There are no words to describe the absolute bliss felt when hard work shows indisputable results.*

Life Lesson #54: *Suffering is an invitation to self-love, self-recognition, and self-healing.*

Life Lesson #55: *Liberate yourself with divine love to better embrace the miracle of all creation.*

Life Lesson #56: *Hope is best served with commitment and action rather than imaginings.*

Life Lesson #57: *Don't talk yourself out of doing something that feeds your spirit, especially with excuses that come automatically.*

Life Lesson #58: *Awaken to the reality that true richness is the gift of life itself!*

Life Lesson #59: *Never doubt that miracles occur.*

Life Lesson #60: *We are ALL miracles placed on this planet to love.*

Life Lesson #61: *If one person can achieve the seemingly impossible,* *every single one of us is in the position to do the same. We are far more likely to realize our heart's desire if we truly believe in possibility.*

Life Lesson #62: *Live life to its fullest; make time for adventure and joy.*

Life Lesson #63: *Do not make excuses; mind, body, and soul must be in concert in order to reach your highest potential.*

Life Lesson #64: *Fear and negativity cripple us, limit us, and keep us from becoming who we were always meant to be.*

Life Lesson #65: *Life is a great adventure—hold on with your heart and savor every instant with sweet appreciation!*

APPENDIX B

Condensed Adaptation: The Warrior's Arsenal: *Twenty-One Weapons for Survival and Victory*

"As I stand in the heart of the drama, surrounded by God's light, I become the master of my fate!"
~JIMMI-ANN

Honing my skills and utilizing the tools that came into my life as a result of *the* cancer journey helped me build a place of safety and resiliency within.

The Power of Prayer
I became aware that prayer is everywhere. I chose to pray for others and asked them to pray for me. The prayers for renewed health were miraculously answered.

Hope and Belief
Never give up! As devastating as the prognosis was, I never gave in to it. I never owned it. I consistently referred to it as *the* cancer and never claimed it. I experienced crushing emotions but obstinately refused to lose hope. Somehow, I held on to the belief that all would be well. I stubbornly refused to go without a fight!

Doubt and Fear

Intuition directed that I could beat *the* cancer if I could relinquish foreboding. Anger, Doubt, Grief, and Fear were constant companions, characters in my life's play. Once able to trust, accept, and welcome them, Doubt, Fear, etc., became insignificant because I chose Love to accompany me on my journey instead.

Uplifting Support of Family and Friends

I embrace the enfolding affection and strength of those close to me—the earthly angels whose compassion lightens my spirit and fuels my determination to survive. My family and friends help me realize that even as I confront Cancer, I can lift my wings and soar! Loving relationships are powerful remedies!

Medicine

I decided to utilize just about every method available to me to combat the dreaded disease. Although I had shortcomings about the effects of chemotherapy wreaking havoc upon my bodily systems, I fought with it as well. Every tool I employed worked harmoniously to facilitate my ultimate recovery.

Healing Foods

Organic whole foods may act as medicine or nourishment in your body, while conventional foods may act as poison. Whenever possible, I choose food wisely because it is integral to the arsenal of healthy living. This lifestyle change was crucial to my recovery, as a modified organic macrobiotic lifestyle, including suggested vitamins and supplements, helped me to win the war against Cancer.

Stress Relief

In searching for unconventional approaches to wellness, I took classes in meditation and sound therapy and saw a hypnotherapist who helped me release fears and achieve profound relaxation. I looked to energy healing, an ancient modality involving the act of moving and shifting energy in the body to support its natural capacity to heal.

The Power of Positivity
The more I focused on staying optimistic, the easier my journey became. I would not be here today if I had dwelt on negativity and the doctor's diagnosis. The more I practiced hopeful thinking, the less troubled I became. I *knew* I had to "get messages" to my subconscious, and working at staying upbeat was an excellent way to begin.

The Advocacy of Words
I learned that I should be cautious in choosing words, especially the words I was thinking, because I realized the negative dialogue echoing inside my head had adversely affected my health. I paid attention to books, texts, song lyrics, and similar resources as they came into my consciousness, and I began to think, speak, and act from a place of greater awareness and understanding.

Say or Sing it Until You Believe It
Consistent repetition of what I wanted to be true was imperative to healing. The more I repeated the outcomes I so desperately desired, the easier believing became. Repetition helped me to manifest healing by connecting to my unconscious thoughts. Acting and singing as if what I wished for had already happened significantly enhanced my recovery.

God-Incidences
Coincidences are more appropriately named, for me, God-Incidences. They became gateways to miracles—opportunities awaiting discovery! I became aware of miracles available for the taking and gratefully rejoiced in accepting them. My advice is to become mindful of the possibilities open to you!

Slowing Down
Forever rushing around in my chaotic world, I learned to slow down and become aware of life itself. This became a most precious gift and also allowed me the time to recognize opportunities and miraculous pathways. Life became more joyous as I learned to live in the present.

Living in the Present
I found the courage to let go of worrying about the past and future. Once I began living in the here and now, life ultimately became joyfully harmonious.

Getting Out in Nature
Mother Earth is a great healer. Sunshine is known for purifying and as an excellent booster of vitamin D. Getting outdoors, reflecting upon its beauty, breathing fresh air, and being grateful for all its glory deliver peace and harmony. Going outside makes one smile and helps relieve anxiety and depression.

The Body in Motion
As bad a shape as I was in, the challenging endeavor of walking ignited an impressive lifestyle change in my fitness level. After years of not exercising, the simple act of getting off the couch and moving was the first step to a healthier life and outlook!

Exercise
After I started my fitness endeavors with walking, life-saving foods gave me significant energy to exercise earnestly. Adding swimming and dancing to my bid for fitness helped me get oxygen to the cellular level, and malignant cells cannot live in an oxygenated environment.

Humor, Chuckles and Grins
Laughter increases endorphins and natural painkillers by getting oxygen deep into the cells. I decided it could help me. I incorporated deep belly laughter into my days to help me deal with *the* Cancer.

Stepping Out—Breaking Out of Self-Imposed Isolation
Getting out into the world became a happy distraction from the disease. Being surrounded by people who cared about me was blessedly gratifying, and I learned not to shut them out in my grief. Stepping out brought normality into my life, allowing me the opportunity to *play*. Confinement or isolation is non-productive and depressing.

Distractive Action
I discovered that focused activity was an essential element of healing. Building, making, creating, and designing let me focus elsewhere while working toward wellness. I endorse it as an excellent method to get one's mind off troubles.

Acceptance and Gratitude
Acceptance and gratitude for *the* cancer allowed the freedom of my body, mind, and soul to repair through the greatest healer—Love.

Love
Love is the most potent and essential tool in the arsenal. Learning to accept myself and to have self-compassion and forgiveness proved crucial to my healing. Through my soul journey, I discovered that I must *love myself completely*. Learning to step into self-love was the gateway, the access point, that allowed me to stand firm in my conviction, grow through adversity, and have absolute faith that I'd win my battle with cancer.

Loving oneself is eye-opening, and it freed me to believe in and accept that unconditional love is the key.

Practicing self-love requires daily attention and intentional action. It demanded that I release old thought patterns and step compassionately into my heart's gracious and abounding wisdom.

RESOURCES

"I am so grateful for these people, their words, and their miracles that provided pathways to my victory!"
~JIMMI-ANN

The Desiderata is a poem written by Max Ehrmann in the early 1920s. The Latin definition of desiderata is "things desired." I was introduced to the work in the 1970s; its message is an archetype for personal evolution, contentment, and joy. It was a guiding beacon during my transformational journey!

Roxanne Koteles-Smith, author of *The Cancer Cookbook, Food for Life*, Author House, 2004, my food coach, and her modified macrobiotic food plan: *FoodWisdomRx*™.

Every Little Cell in My Body is Happy and Well is a song Unity Church uses to promote physical and mental wellness. It is sung to the tune of Stephen Foster's 'Shortnin' Bread,' and a church official told me that Wally Amos penned the lyrics. (My research did not uncover definitive answers about the song.)

Singing it was elemental to my recovery because it helped me 'get messages' deep into my cells that I was healthy! It became music therapy as I frequently sang it; the repetition of the melody and rhythm stimulated positive brain performance. I used the song to help pull me from survival mode and anxiety to relaxation, calmness, and belief. I suggest you go to the internet and find this song to help you achieve well-being.

Frames of Mind: The Theory of Multiple Intelligences, Basic Books, 2011, was first presented by Howard Granger in this 1983 volume. He proposed that people have different ways of being smart and that traditional methods of looking at and measuring intelligence are too restrictive. His theory supports nine ways people can be smart: linguistic-verbal, logical-mathematical, visual-spatial, bodily-kinesthetic, musical, interpersonal, intrapersonal, naturalistic, and existentialistic intelligences. Camperdown Academy uses his approach to better prepare our middle school students for the rigors of high school.

Amenie Kristine Schweizer, my friend, is a Certified Holistic Health Practitioner with an emphasis on supporting others using integrative and transformational tools, including life coaching, energetic healing, and aromatherapy. She was also instrumental as she became my writing coach after I *thought* the book was completed.

Laughter Yoga International https://www.laughteryoga.org/ Laughter Yoga International is a global movement for better health and happiness; it fosters world peace through voluntary laughter. Laughter Yoga (LY) is an exercise program practiced in more than 110 countries and was developed by Dr. Madan Kataria, an Indian medical doctor who chose to help people get well with deep belly chuckles. LY incorporates its laughter exercises with yogic breathing techniques. It is a system that provokes laughter without depending upon humor, jokes, or comedy. Through LY exercises, genuine, spontaneous laughter occurs, bringing more oxygen to the brain and making one feel more energetic and healthier! LY exercising for ten minutes or longer adds oxygen to your cells to reduce stress, enhances the immune system, and helps thoughts remain positive during challenging experiences.

Miracles, Hay House, 2008, by Stuart Wilde was one of the most essential and inspiring bits of information revealed to me during my journey. Wilde professes that when we believe that the 'living spirit of love' resides within, miracles are ours for the taking. I adapted his *'Understanding the Nature of Beliefs'* from the book as my 'Wellness Plan' to guide me as I navigated the path of my evolutionary journey. His words were exactly what I needed, for I have always believed that part of the living spirit of God lives in everyone and everything.

The Hidden Messages in Water, Atria Books, 2004, by Masaru Emoto, a Japanese researcher, revealed vital information to my recovery. Emoto conducted tests on water that convinced me that my thoughts affect everything in and around me—his experiments profoundly changed my life. This information inspired me to stop the negative dialogue in my head and hold myself in high esteem, permitting healing to begin.

What the Bleep Do We Know!?, directed by, William Artz, Betty Chase, and Mark Vicente, is a 2004 documentary/drama merging quantum physics with a storyline illustrating that everything is related—nothing stands alone. It proposes that there is a soul connection between quantum physics and cognizance. It suggests that we create our world with our thoughts, and I was determined to generate my world as cancer-free!

Steve Harrison's *Get Published Now* Course and the entire AuthorSuccess.com team. For technical help & support. Bradley Communications Corp, 390 Reed Road, Broomall, Pennsylvania 19008, United States.

ENDNOTES

"The end is actually the beginning . . . "
~JIMMI-ANN

1. Roxanne Koteles-Smith, *The Cancer Cookbook: Food for Life*, Bloomington, IN: Author House, 2004.
2. FoodWisdomrx™, https://FoodWisdomrx.com.
3. "Celiac disease - Symptoms and causes," Mayo Clinic, last modified August 10, 2021. https://www.mayoclinic.org/diseases-conditions/celiac-disease/symptoms-causes/syc-20352220.
4. Greg Timmons, "Hippocrates," Biography, last modified August 9, 2023. https://www.biography.com/scholars-educators/hippocrates.
5. Laura Dolson, "The importance of Phytonutrients for Your Health," Verywell Fit, last modified June 3, 2022 https://www.verywellfit.com/phytonutrients-phytochemicals-2242002.
6. "Can Deep Breathing Be Key to Cancer Healing? You Bet!" Hope4Cancer, last modified September 21, 2015 https://hope4cancer.com/blog/can-deep-breathing-be-key-to-cancer-healing-you-bet/.//.
7. Janelle Ringer, "Laughter: A Fool-Proof Prescription," Loma Linda University Health website, last modified, April 1, 2021 https://news.llu.edu/research/laughter-fool-proof-prescription.
8. William Arntz, Betsy Chase, Mark Vincent, *What the Bleep Do We Know?!* Portland, Oregon: Captured Light and Lord of the Wind, 2004.
9. Masaru Emoto, *The Hidden Messages in Water* (New York: Simon and Schuster, 2005).
10. Stuart Wilde, *Miracles* (Carlsbad, CA: Hay House, 2007).

11. Jaime Herndon, "What are the Benefits and Risks of a Chemotherapy Port?" Healthline, last modified May 27, 2021, https://www.healthline.com/health/cancer/chemotherapy-port.
12. K. Adams, M. Kohlmeier, M. Powell, and S.H. Zeisel, "Nutrition in Medicine," 2010, American Society for Parenteral and Enteral Nutrition, last modified October 20, 2010, https://doi.org/10.1177/0884533610379606.
13. "PET scan, Positron emission topography," Mayo Clinic, last modified April 18, 2023, https://www.mayoclinic.org/tests-procedures/pet-scan/about/pac-20385078.
14. "MRI," Mayo Clinic, last modified September 9, 2023. https://www.mayoclinic.org/test-procedures/mri/about/pac-20384768

ACKNOWLEDGMENTS

"Thank you, thank you, thank you—my heart overflows with grateful acknowledgment to the stellar supporting cast that accompanied me on my triumphant transformational journey and the cast of thousands who helped bring this manuscript to the press!"
~JIMMI-ANN

Thank you, again, to my incredible cast of characters who have already been recognized in the book. I am also grateful to my *first readers* and all the doctors, nurses, and staff who took great care of me.

Additionally, I appreciate the exceptionally creative team with Steve Harrison Publishing & Bradley Communications: Steve Harrison, Mary Lou Reed, Sheri Horn Hasan, Christy Day, Kim Cruise, Cristina Smith, Maggie McLaughlin, Joe McAllister, Valerie Costa, Geoffrey Berwind, Debby Englander, Sarah Brown, Veronica Karaman, Trish Roberts, Lynn Tramonte, Darity Wesley.

Thank you to Barbara Shaw Binson for the amazing photography.

Thank you to our families and extended families: Carnes, Seeger, Grey, Jester, Davis, Hall, Richey, Brown, Brinson, Schweizer, Ellison, Bowers, Porter, Baldwin, Rios, Pindroh, Coburn, McMillian, DuPuy, Mease. Deborah, Claude, Claude Austin, Paula, Joe, Anna, Justin, Jordan, James, Debra, Matthew, Jordan, Connie, James, Kevin, Sarah, D.J., Emilie, Audrey, Lisa Marie, Tracy, Gail Bowers, Casey, and Chris. Thank you to my granddaughter, Trina Jester for creative support.

Cheers to Roxanne Koteles, Gary and Kathy Ellison, Dr. and Mrs. Ronald Grisanti, Rosie Koteles-Halapin, Stephen Corso, Paige Turner, Dr. Roseanne Diehl, Dr. Milner, Dr. and Mrs. Ronald Grisanti, Kay Hart, Candy and Frank, Angie Holt Grech, Beth Holcombe Issac, Jeanne Dove, Kathleen Carey, Donna Mease, Monica Kemp, Erin Leopold.

A special thank you to *all* of the Camperdown Academy *family, faculty, staff, students, and their families past and present* – including Pat Porter, Meg Coffey, Virginia Meador, Pat Golus, Linda Grant, Linda Stone, Susan McLeod, Dana Blackhurst, William Van Cleeve, Heidi Bishop, Ruth Benson, Elliot Stewart, Nona Cheek, Maxine Bennett, Amy Brooke, Angie Buchanan, Jeremy Bullinger, Diana Carey, Myrtie Carter, Jane Chang, Karin Chickvary, Stephen Cook, Debi Fisher, Thayer Fleming, Dewa Greenleaf, Barbara Guryan, Tiffany Jones DuPuy, Mara Lasater, Sherrill Livernois, Susan Newton, Courtney Stefanik, Susan Reiner, Millie Runion, Lauren Schuessler Hunt, Cathy Westbrook, Ben Shiley, Suzanna Greer, Dan Blanch, Daniel Nichols, Anne Copeland, Chana Fletcher, Sarah Lynch, and RECT (Retired Excellent Camperdown Teachers.)

Gratitude to: Outer Banks friends and *Lost Colony* Fossils, including Amenie Schweizer, Mary and Le Hook, Jim Fineman, Sissy Gaskins, Wayne Garish, Kennetha Parker-Howes and Dancy, and the Pony Island Restaurant for carefully cooking my organic meals!

Hugs to Lisa, Allen Wells, and family, also to Trish, Tony, and Elijah Tucker, Anita, John, Kenny, Heather, Kevin, Keith, Landy, Zach, Martha, Patty and Thomas Quiroz, Carlos, Sylvia and Fernando Arango, Norma Joiner, Andrea Velez, Marianna Velez, Laura Salazar.

"Bravo!" to The Greenville Theater, Allen and Suzanne McCalla, Charlie Miller, Kimberlee Ferreira, and the extraordinarily supportive cast, crew, and staff of *Hello, Dolly!* Harriet Brewington, Anne Gibson, the *Dollies*, and the wonderful audience members!

A fond thank you to my comforting friends, Buzz, Grace, Gemma, and Gomer!

"Please forgive me if my sometimes-inefficient intellectual instrument failed to list you individually for your exquisite role in my recovery! I will suddenly remember hundreds of other names after this goes to print... you were temporarily misplaced! Thank you for your contributions to my *wonderful life!*"
~JIMMI-ANN

GET TO KNOW THE AUTHOR

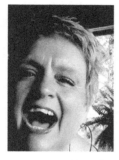

Jimmi-Ann Carnes Muse is an author, playwright, actor, educator, visual artist, and motivational speaker. *Stage 4 to Center Stage!* is her first book; it offers optimism and hope in the face of the darkest diagnoses. She adopted established and unconventional approaches to defeat terminal cancer and hopes her success urges others to do the same.

She is a master teacher with forty-one years of experience teaching theater arts, playwriting, Shakespeare, language arts, language dramatics, visual arts, and Multiple Intelligences. She also facilitates Laughter Yoga and SoulCollage® workshops; she enjoys various art forms, especially stained glass, watercolors, and jewelry making.

Jimmi-Ann lives in South Carolina with David, her husband, and their tabby cat, Gomer, who rescued them. Jimmi-Ann has always enjoyed writing and authored countless plays for her young actors to perform during her teaching career. Family is of the utmost importance to the couple, and happily, their children, grandchildren, and great-grandchildren *all* live nearby.

Renowned for her larger-than-life personality and wonderfully infectious laughter, her most sincere wish is for her readers to understand: *If one person can achieve the seemingly impossible, every one of us is in the position to do the same. We are likely to realize our heart's desire if we truly believe in possibility.*

"Laughs With Great Thunder" is a nickname given to me by a colleague since I am known for my echoing laughter!

**"Break-a-leg!
I love you!"**

~ JIMMI-ANN

Made in the USA
Middletown, DE
07 March 2024